WALKING RX

BENEFITS OF WALKING

Dr. R. Ahmed

Disclaimer and Legal Notice

Dedication

This book is dedicated to all those who live a sedentary lifestyle especially those who spend countless long hours working at their desks.

Acknowledgement

I want to thank God (for answering my prayers when most needed), my wife, Dr. Saleema, (for being a pillar of strength in times of weakness), my sons Zeeshan & Faizan (for being the 'why' in my life), my parents Nasir & Dr. Safia (for teaching me resilience) and last but not least, my readers for taking the time to not only read my material but also for providing valuable feedback, inspiration, and motivation which encourages me to become a better writer and to provide high-quality content. Thank you!

Table of Contents

Introduction

With its long list of positive effects and negligible downsides, walking is the gold standard of physical activity. It's hassle-free (imagine that—no tools required!) and there are only a small number of diseases and conditions where it shouldn't be used. You could question if there are benefits for everyone since it's an exercise that can help someone in their nineties maintain their fitness. Yes, with the correct tactics, people of all ages and fitness levels, from complete beginners to elite-level athletes, may reap many of the same benefits from walking workouts as they would from running. When people think of healthy habits, they automatically think of Pilates, yoga, and the trusty old treadmill. However, walking is the more understated workout that has all the benefits but has yet to receive the media hype.

Walking is an excellent kind of exercise for beginners. Since it is free, easy, and available to everyone, walking is the ideal kind of physical activity. You don't need anything fancy or a certain degree of fitness, and you can do it just about anywhere. The advantages are vast, ranging from better physical health to enhanced emotional well-being. There is no required degree of fitness for walking. When should one consider walking to be exercise, as opposed to taking a few steps here and there to throw some laundry in the dryer or fetch something to eat from the kitchen? These kinds of steps, in addition to the steps you take during a targeted walk (such as a thirty-minute stroll through your neighborhood or an afternoon trek), are beneficial to your general health and should be taken whenever possible. According to Amanda Paluch, PhD, an assistant professor at the University of Massachusetts in Amherst who specializes in the study of physical activity epidemiology and kinesiology, "all steps, regardless of intensity, count toward our physical activity and have the potentialto have positive effects on our health". (Although variables such as pace and the steepness of an incline can certainly make some steps more taxing) (Asp et al., 2022).

Walking falls into the category of aerobic exercise with moderate intensity when you walk at a pace that causes your breathing to become slightly more rapid (although you should still be able to have a conversation while walking at this pace). The American College of Sports Medicine recommends that individuals get at least 150 minutes per week of moderate physical activity. Thisequates to a total of five sessions each week, consisting of thirty minutes each. Even though thirty minutes is the recommended amount of time for a walk, Dr. I-Min Lee, a professor of medicine at Harvard Medical School, recommends beginning with three shorter walks of ten minutes each and gradually increasing the length of your walks until you reach thirty minutes once you feel comfortable doing so *(Put Your Best Foot Forward: Why Walking Is Good for You, 2014)*. The Centers for Disease Control and Prevention (CDC) suggest that individuals obtain at least 150 minutes of this type of activity per week to boost cardiovascular health and lessen the risk of other chronic diseases. It is important to remember that engaging in more physical activity is often associated with experiencing a greater number of positive health effects. That means that if you walk at a difficult enough pace to make it a moderate-intensity activity, you can satisfy the recommendation for cardiovascular exercise by walking for five sessions of thirty minutes each, five times each week. If you get started right away, you'll begin to see positive changes in both yourmind and your body in a short amount of time. According to estimates provided by the National Health Service (NHS), a personwho weighs 60 kilograms (9.5 stone) and walks for just thirty minutes will burn 99 calories. This is a significant contribution to weight loss *(Put Your Best Foot Forward: Why Walking Is Good for You, 2014)*.

On the other hand, according to Dr. Paluch, whose study focuses on the health advantages of daily step counts, there are no official recommendations for how many steps to take per day. Some research suggests that merely 7,500 steps per day may be a more meaningful threshold for improved health. Even though the widespread recommendation is to strive to take 10,000 steps per day, this recommendation is based on very little scientific data (Asp et al., 2022).

While walking is a wonderful activity for maintaining one's health and fitness, to derive the maximum benefit from this activity, one must walk in the correct manner. You may argue that everybody walks, yet there is a proper technique for walking to get exercise. If you want to get the most out of walking as a form of exercise, you should focus on maintaining correct posture and technique. The cardiovascular and muscular benefits of walking can be increased by engaging the core muscles, maintaining an upright position, and taking longer steps. In addition, increasing the intensity of this straightforward yet potent exercise by integrating intervals of rapid walking or adding ankle weights will significantly boost both the intensity and efficiency of the workout. You should obviously be aware of any potential dangers that may lie in your way; nevertheless, you should direct your focus a few feet in front of you rather than directly at your own feet. Allow your arms to swing freely and roll your weight through the sole of your foot, moving from heel to toe.

Before beginning a new fitness routine, it is essential to discuss the matter with your primary care physician, particularly if you suffer from a persistent health issue such as asthma or heart disease. Walking can also make other disorders, such as osteoarthritis in the spine or knee injuries, much worse. Before beginning a walking fitness routine, it is important to discuss the matter with your primary care physician, particularly if you have a history of injuries or other persistent health conditions that could be exacerbated by the activity. Your doctor will be able to evaluate your unique situation and provide direction regarding whether walking is appropriate for you, as well as whether or not there are any adjustments you should make. They might also suggest other forms of physical activity that are better suited to your requirements and restrictions than the ones you've been doing.

Always remember that it is best to err on the side of caution and seek the counsel of a professional to safeguard your safety and well-being while engaging in physical activity. Many of the health challenges that have plagued the populace can be effectively rolled back with a regime of walking. In a report by Public Health England in 2017, it was reported that almost one in four (22.4%) ofthe English population is defined as 'inactive' by virtue of doing less than 30 minutes of activity per week and has the highest riskof ill health due to insufficient physical activity (England, 2017).

When you embark on walking, you unveil a treasure trove of wonder that you may never have imagined. As simple as walking is, which is often dismissed by many as not a serious enough exercise, each step tells a story—a captivating one—that reveals hidden rewards and concealed advantages. Come with me and let us walk the pages of this book together. As we tread the path of revelation, you'll find that the benefits of walking extend far beyond what you might have initially thought. Fear not, for this expedition shall not be cut short; we shall journey hand in hand tillthe very last page, where the tapestry of proven walking benefits shall be laid bare, a testament to the extraordinary power of putting one foot in front of the other.

CHAPTER ONE

Getting Started

The allure of walking benefits, though enchanting, might seemalmost fantastical, causing an immediate urge to dive in. It's a siren's call to wellness and vitality that's hard to resist; yet, amid this eagerness, pause for a moment, for I have a tale to weave; a tale of embarking on this journey with knowledge and strategy, ensuring that every stride is a step towards optimal gains.As in any grand expedition, a path paved with intentionality yields the richest rewards. So, as you prepare to embrace the rhythm of your footsteps, remember that this venture requires more than justthe act of walking itself. There's an art to the inception and a method to the movement that guarantees a fulfilling odyssey. The journey begins not only with that initial step but also with an understanding of the nuances that lie beneath the surface of this seemingly simple act. Delve deeper with me, and I shall unravel the secrets to begin this journey on the right foot. Much like a symphony, walking has its own notes and rhythms. It's a dance between your body and the earth, a dialogue between muscles and momentum. To make the most of this partnership, consider the following as your prelude to the magnificent symphony of strides that awaits.

Right footwear

Since your leg is going to be the primary instrument that you use for this workout, it is only natural that you begin there. Invest in a pair of shoes that will make walking easier for you. Try on your prospective walking shoes with the socks that you intend to use throughout your workout, and do it at the end of the day, when your feet will be slightly swollen from the day's activities. Both factors can have a significant impact on the way a pair of shoes fits on the foot. Keep an eye out for footwear designed specifically for walking. Because our heels are part of our feet that make contact with the ground first when we walk, the majority of shoes designed specifically for walking feature an Achilles notch, which is a little depression in the back of the shoe that helps ease the stress on the Achilles tendon. It is essential that the toe box provides enough space for your toes to wiggle and that the heel of the shoe not slide around. You should also look for a shoe that is lightweight, has ventilation, and has a sole that has some degree of flexibility so that it can move with your foot.

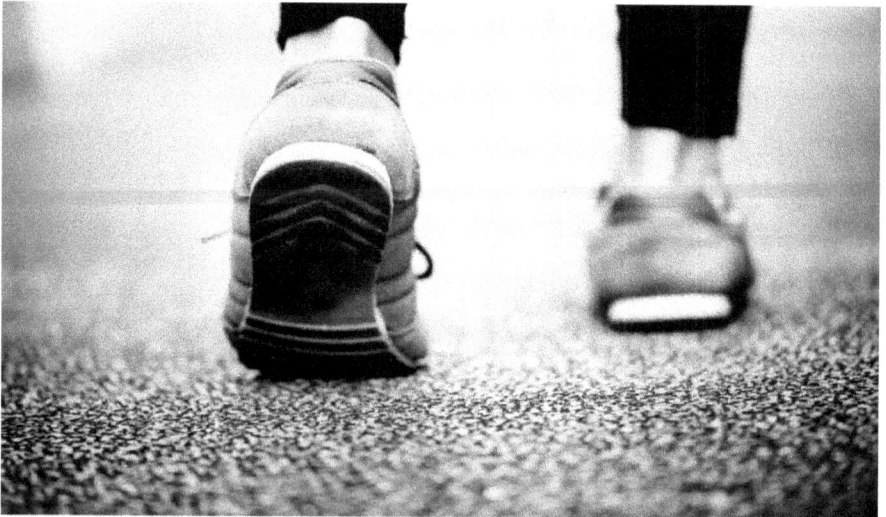

Clothing

When it comes to your wardrobe, opt for comfortable textiles that allow air to circulate, such as cotton, and dress in layers. If you do start to feel warm, you will be able to take off a layer, wrap it around your waist, or carry it with you for the remainder of your walk. This way, you can easily maintain a comfortable body temperature throughout your walk. Additionally, choosing breathable fabrics like linen or bamboo can also help keep you cooland prevent excessive sweating.

Plan your route

If you have never gone for a walk before, you should look for a spot where you can make short loops, since this will enable you toreturn to your starting position on multiple occasions. This gives you the opportunity to reassess your capabilities as well as listen toyour body. You have the motivation to go another lap based on what you are feeling in your body; it's a little mind game on your body when you consider how quickly you finished a lap. Do not putstress on yourself by going on these long treks right away at the beginning of the game. There will be times when you go five minutes without speaking, and that is perfectly normal. The best approach to getting in touch with nature is to go for a walk. You have the option of taking the path that takes you through the forest(green). Walking through green areas has been shown to lower stress levels, improve mental health, and improve physical health, according to the findings of a research team from Essex University called Green Exercise.

Pick a suitable pace

Paying attention to how quickly you walk might be a significant factor in determining whether or not it counts as a workout. Some beginners start off at a pace that is too fast for them to maintain after a few days; this is a mistake that you should steer clear of at all costs. It is more sustainable to set a pace that you are comfortable with and then raise your tempo (speed) as you progress in your walking ability. It is not a good idea to choose a pace that requires you to walk so slowly, either, because the benefits to your cardiovascular system will be minimal as a result.

Walking at a brisk pace is the most effective way to increase fitness; the pace at which you consider walking to be "brisk" will depend on your present level of fitness. It is normal for your breathing to become more labored as you walk quickly; nevertheless, you should still be able to carry on a conversation.

The arrow pointing right and up means that when you are out of breath and unable to carry on a conversation with the person next to you, it is time to slow down. The following are some suggestions on how to walk briskly:

- Beginning at a leisurely pace will allow you to warm up, and continuing at that pace will allow you to cool down.

- Keeping the shoulders relaxed and down, while keeping the back long and straight, is essential.

- From the back of the heel, roll the foot forward.

- If a person's feet are hurting after going for a fast walk, giving their feet a massage, or bathing them in warm water may help alleviate the discomfort.

Schedule your walk

Walking is likely something you do on a daily basis; you shouldn't make it a regular part of your fitness routine. Walking experts recommend setting aside at least one day of the week for rest and relaxation. You have the option of taking a full recuperation day where you do not engage in any form of physical activity, going for a short stroll in a relaxed manner, planning a day of cross-training in which you, for instance, ride your bike at a leisurely speed, etc.

Here is a walking workout schedule sample for newbies that can take you from Day 1 through Week 12 and into a new healthy lifestyle! This walking program's end goal is for you to be able to walk for thirty to sixty minutes, five to seven days each week (Pollard, 2022).

12 Week Sample Walking Program

	WARM UP	ACTIVITY (Target Zone*)	COOL DOWN	TOTAL TIME	PROGRESS ☑
WEEK 1 3x/week (Alternate days)	Walk Slowly 5 min.	Walk Briskly 5 min.	Walk Slowly 5 min.	15 min.	☐☐☐
WEEK 2 3x/week	Walk Slowly 5 min.	Walk Briskly 7 min.	Walk Slowly 5 min.	17 min.	☐☐☐
WEEK 3 3x/week	Walk Slowly 5 min.	Walk Briskly 9 min.	Walk Slowly 5 min.	19 min.	☐☐☐
WEEK 4 3x/week	Walk Slowly 5 min.	Walk Briskly 11 min.	Walk Slowly 5 min.	21 min.	☐☐☐
WEEK 5 4x/week	Walk Slowly 5 min.	Walk Briskly 13 min.	Walk Slowly 5 min.	23 min.	☐☐☐☐
WEEK 6 4x/week	Walk Slowly 5 min.	Walk Briskly 15 min.	Walk Slowly 5 min.	25 min.	☐☐☐☐
WEEK 7 4x/week	Walk Slowly 5 min.	Walk Briskly 18 min.	Walk Slowly 5 min.	28 min.	☐☐☐☐
WEEK 8 4x/week	Walk Slowly 5 min.	Walk Briskly 20 min.	Walk Slowly 5 min.	30 min.	☐☐☐☐
WEEK 9 5x/week	Walk Slowly 5 min.	Walk Briskly 23 min.	Walk Slowly 5 min.	33 min.	☐☐☐☐☐
WEEK 10 5x/week	Walk Slowly 5 min.	Walk Briskly 26 min.	Walk Slowly 5 min.	36 min.	☐☐☐☐☐
WEEK 11 5x/week	Walk Slowly 5 min.	Walk Briskly 28 min.	Walk Slowly 5 min.	38 min.	☐☐☐☐☐
WEEK 12 5x/week	Walk Slowly 5 min.	Walk Briskly 30 min.	Walk Slowly 5 min.	40 min.	☐☐☐☐☐

*As you improve your fitness, try to walk within the upper range of your target heart rate zone.

(Adapted from National Heart, Lung, and Blood Institute[2] and University of Wisconsin School of Medicine and Pubic Health[3])

People of varying fitness levels can find that walking is a tough kind of exercise to engage in. Nevertheless, not everyone will find the same kinds of walks to be tough. Increase the pressure by utilizing these several tactics.

- **Climb some steep slopes on foot**. Find a hilly path to walk on so that you can improve your strength and stamina or perform hill repeats by going up and down the same hill multiple times in succession. Remember a few pointers about proper form. When going uphill, experts recommend that you walk with a small forward lean. In addition, because walking downhill can be taxing on the knees, you should walk more slowly, take shorter steps, and keep your knees bent over a little.

- **Train at intervals:** Interval training consists of alternating bouts of high-intensity labor and lower-intensity recuperation intervals. First, walk as quickly as you can during the specified amount of time, and then gradually slow down. You could, for example, walk at a normal pace for two or three minutes and then walk very quickly for one minute. This would be one example. Alternate between walking quickly for one minute and walking slowly for the following minute for an easier option. You can use visible markers such as trees or poles and increase your speed between every fourth and fifth tree or pole. If using a clock is too inconvenient a method, utilize these visible markers instead.

- **Change your terrain:** Pavement is invariably a fantastic option, but you should also explore using different types of surfaces. Walking on grass or gravel can help you burn more calories than walking on a track does. The bonus? You can boost the number of calories you burn by walking on the sand if you happen to live near the ocean.

Keep yourself hydrated.

Be sure to drink a lot of water before going out, even if you'll only be walking for a short amount of time, since this will help you stay hydrated during your walk. If you are going to be walking for more than half an hour, though, you should bring a bottle of water with you so that you can sip on it while you are walking. You should aim to consume between a half cup and a full cup of water for every mile that you cover while walking. If you are going on a long walk, it is helpful to know this information so that you can plan how much water to bring with you.

Invite Friends

The best part about going for a walk is that you can do it byyourself or with others, and it won't cost you a dime. It is always more fun to participate in activities with friends or coworkers.Invite the people in your social circle to accompany you on your walk. If you have the opportunity, you could challenge them to a "walk-off." Competition spices things up. You can keep yourself motivated to continue improving your walking time by including some healthy competition in your walking regimen. You can meet people who share your interests and interact with them during your walk-off by using one of the many applications that are available on the internet. This will also make it easier for you to track your development and compete against previous versions of yourself. Your ability to experience a sense of community will make it easier for you to incorporate walking into your daily life. And interacting with new individuals is not a prerequisite for having social relationships; it may mean bringing along a pet with you on your daily walk.

Stay Motivated

You are the number one fan of your desire for the healthy lifestyle that walking provides. The flames of your motivation must never waver, for there will inevitably come mornings when the allure of cocooning in warm sheets seems irresistible, tempting you to stray from the path you've chosen. Yet, let these moments be reminders of your commitment to yourself. Remember, even the most skilled conductor requires motivation. Keep your aspirations at the forefront of your consciousness, like cherished notes in a composition, and scatter them strategically throughout yourabode. Let your dwelling be adorned with gentle nudges towards your goals—a visual tapestry of your journey towards an invigorating life. Your commitment to a healthy lifestyle issacrosanct and not subject to compromise or negotiation. It's not merely a desire, but a testament to your tenacity.

Though the applause of a crowd may be absent, you must step into the spotlight of self-encouragement. Become the maestro of your motivation and the conductor of your own cheers. In the grand theater of life, you are both the performer and the audience. Rally your own spirits with a resounding call to action. You are not just a follower of a healthier lifestyle; you are its most ardent advocate and its true embodiment. The journey is yours to embrace, and with each step, you reaffirm your status as the unwavering champion of your vibrant desires. A healthy lifestyle is not up for negotiation; if no one cheers you on, be your own cheerleader!

Walking or running—which is better?

Walking has the same health benefits as running. To start, let's get one thing out of the way: Neither one is "better" than the other. It all boils down to the fitness goals you have and the capabilities of your body. Because they do not have as much time as other people do to get a workout in, several individuals choose to run the distance of four miles rather than walk it. It is not a question of which alternative is preferable because the answer depends on your purpose; therefore, you cannot compare the two.

Walking is a great option for getting into shape, so it's a wonderful alternative for people who are just starting out with fitness. In a similar vein, it is the least intimidating kind of physical activity for first timers. Walking is one of the best forms of exercise since it has the lowest dropout rate of all the different types of exercise. This is one of the best aspects of choosing walking as your form of exercise. This is due to the fact that you are required to walk every day regardless, so there is no way to really avoid it.

Keep in mind that you are creating your masterpiece as you step onto the new canvas that each day presents to you. Take responsibility for your own well-being and allow your doggedness to serve as the cornerstone of your ascent to greatness. Bring your goals to life by imagining a brighter future with each new daybreak. Walking is the key to a better lifestyle, and now is the perfect time to start uncovering all of the many benefits that walking can provide.

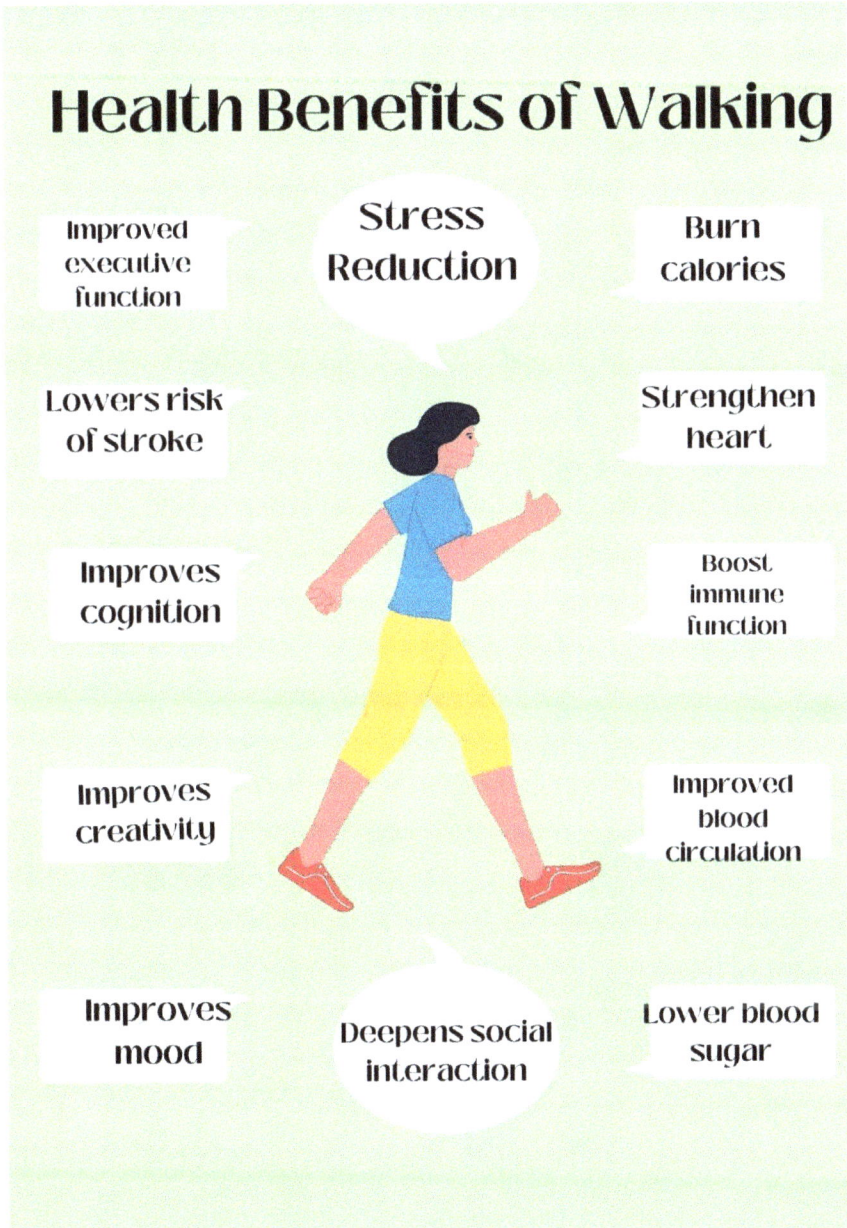

Health Benefits of Walking

Improved executive function

Stress Reduction

Burn calories

Lowers risk of stroke

Strengthen heart

Improves cognition

Boost immune function

Improves creativity

Improved blood circulation

Improves mood

Deepens social interaction

Lower blood sugar

CHAPTER TWO

Memory

Anna sat at her cluttered desk, surrounded by stacks of papers and a relentless blinking cursor on her computer screen. The weight of deadlines and expectations bore down on her, suffocating her creativity. She pushed her chair back and stood up abruptly, announcing to her colleagues, "I need a walk to clear my head." Anna stepped out into the vibrant city streets, the cacophony of honking horns and chattering pedestrians instantly washing over her. As she walked, her thoughts were jumbled, much like the hustle and bustle around her. She wandered aimlessly, allowing her feet to guide her. Soon, she found herself in a park, where a gentle breeze rustled the leaves and the distant laughter of childrenplaying echoed. She sank onto a bench, closed her eyes, and inhaled deeply. Slowly, the chaos in her mind began to unravel. The scent of blooming flowers and the distant hum of a river calmed her racing heart. With each step, Anna felt her thoughts settle. She noticed the intricate patterns of leaves, the way the sunlight danced through the branches, and the tranquility of nature embracing her. Ideas flowed back, one after another, like a stream finding its course. Returning to her desk, Anna felt rejuvenated. She attacked her work with newfound clarity, inspired by the serenity she had found in her walk. From that day on, she understood the power of stepping away and allowing the world's rhythm to guide her thoughts and renew her spirit.

The story of Anna sheds light on a common practice that many of us engage in if we find that we are unable to think clearly or recall specific information. Could there be a link between getting some exercise and the brain's ability to free itself of a "jamming network"? What is going on "up there" that we cannot see? What connection, if any, is there between walking and memory?

Improves Memory

Memory, in its most basic form, refers to the ongoing process of the retention of knowledge over time. Memory is an essential component of human cognition due to the fact that it enables humans to recall and draw upon experiences from their past in order to form the basis of their understanding of and behavior in the present. Memory also provides people with a framework through which they can make sense of what is happening now and what will happen in the future. As a consequence of this, memory plays a significant role in the process of development. When a new memory is formed, information travels from the cortex, the region of the brain that is densely packed with nerve cells, to the hippocampus, the area of the brain that serves as the primary hub for switching between memories. When we recover a memory, the information travels in the opposite direction from how it was stored.

Walking enhances connections within and between three of the brain's networks, including one that is related to Alzheimer's disease, according to a new study from the University of Maryland School of Public Health. This finding adds to the growing body of evidence that suggests exercise is beneficial to brain health. The research compared the brains and the ability to recall stories of older people who had normal brain function to those who had been diagnosed with mild cognitive impairment. Mild cognitive impairment refers to a minor reduction in mental functions such as memory, logic, and judgment, and it is a risk factor for Alzheimer's disease. The study looked at the brains of older adults who had normal brain function.

"Historically, the brain networks we studied in this research show deterioration over time in people with mild cognitive impairment and Alzheimer's disease," said J. Carson Smith, a kinesiology professor with the School of Public Health and principal investigator of the study. "They become disconnected, and as a result, people lose their ability to think clearly and remember things. We're demonstrating that exercise training strengthens these connections." (*Study Finds Brain Connectivity and Memory Improve in Older Adults After Walking*, 2023) Thirty-three volunteers, ranging in age from 71 to 85 years old, were monitored as they walked for a total of twelve weeks on a treadmill on a daily, four-times-per-week basis. Before and after going through this exercise routine, the researchers had the volunteers read a brieftale and then retell it aloud, trying to include as many specifics as they could remember. Functional magnetic resonance imaging, or fMRI, was also performed on the participants so that the researchers could detect changes in communication both within and between the three brain networks that influence cognitive function. After a period of 12 weeks of exercise, the researchers repeated the tests and discovered that the participant's ability to recall the stories had significantly improved.

WALKING IMPROVES MEMORY

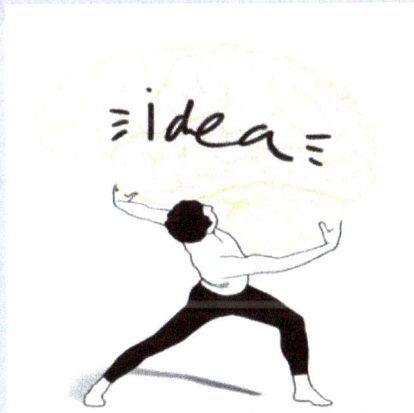

Reverses the effects of aging on brain cells

Around the age of 30, your body naturally begins to lose muscular mass and bone density, and around the age of 40, your brain begins to lose volume to the tune of around 5 percent every decade. This information was provided by Becky Upham in an article that was published on everydayhealth.com on July 19, 2021. The ability to retain a piece of knowledge, such as a password or street name, for an extended period of time, known as working memory, may begin to deteriorate in our thirties, according to some research. At least in terms of your brain, however, according to the findings of a recent study conducted by researchers at Colorado State University, it appears that you may be able to reverse the effects of aging. The participants in the study who went on frequent brisk walks for the duration of the study experienced more improvements in white matter and memory than those who engaged in stretching and balancing exercises for the same period of time. This was in comparison to those who engaged in stretching and balance activities (Upham, 2021).

The purpose of this study was to investigate whether or not regular physical activity has the capability of preventing cognitive decline and fostering good changes in the brain, a phenomenon known as neural plasticity. The focus of the research is on white matter, an area of the brain that has received relatively little attention yet is crucial for typical brain function since it includes nerve fibers. The purpose of this study is to establish whether or not aerobic exercise has the ability to halt or perhaps reverse the deterioration of white matter associated with healthy aging as well as dementia. Participants in the study were divided into groups and required to attend meetings three times per week for a period of six months. During these meetings, one group went on brisk walks lasting forty minutes, another group engaged in supervised stretching and balance training, and a third group learned and practiced choreographed dances. The imaging and testing of the patient's brain were repeated after the completion of the intervention.

Only in the walking group were the alterations in white matter related to improved memory. This was the case for all of the groups. This reveals that when people become more physically active, their white matter, which links and supports the cells in ourbrains, actually remodels itself. On the other hand, white matter has a tendency to tear and shrink in those who lead a sedentary lifestyle. These findings highlight the dynamic nature of our brains and the way in which they are continually transforming themselves, both for the better and for the worse, in response to how we live and move. According to the authors of the study, it is unknown why the dancers did not see the same benefits as the other participants, but it is possible that it is because they were receiving coaching and did not move as aggressively throughout their sessions. It's possible that this indicates that the advantages of white matter were mostly driven by the effects of aerobic activity. According to Andrea Mendez Colmenares, a cognitive neuroscience PhD student at Colorado State University in FortCollins, Colorado, and the lead author of the study, the fact that this study was a randomized controlled trial as opposed to an observational study is one of the things that sets it apart from other studies. The majority of randomized controlled trials that investigate the positive effects of exercise rely on participants reporting on the activities they are already undertaking, which can lead to less credible conclusions.

Reduces brain-damaging stress

Memory, attention, and cognitive flexibility are all negatively impacted by prolonged and repeated exposure to stressful events.It has been proven to be particularly beneficial for reducing stress levels to go for a walk in the great outdoors. According to Andrew Huberman, a neuroscientist in the Department of Neurobiology at Stanford Medicine, the influence of being outside may have something to do with "optic flow," which is the feeling that objects are going past us as we walk. This perception quiets the circuits responsible for stress, and being outside may have something to dowith how "optic flow" works.

"Self-generated optic flow," which may be achieved by activities such as walking, jogging, or cycling, "shifts the brain into a state of relaxation that isn't seen when you're stationary," he explains. Researchers have shown that walking lowers levels of the stress hormone cortisol, which normally rises in response to a perceived threat. According to a review of studies that was published in Frontiers in Aging Neuroscience in 2019, elevated levels of cortisol may be harmful to cognition and contribute to the development of Alzheimer's disease. It has been found that even a short walk of twenty minutes can help relieve stress (*5 Ways Walking Can Boost Your Brain Health*, 2023).

CHAPTER THREE

Walking and Creativity

~⌒

Walking increases creative creativity, according to researchers at Stanford. People's levels of inventiveness were compared between those who were sitting and those who were walking. Walking increased an individual's creative output by 60% on average.

According to a research co-authored by Professor Daniel Schwartz of the Stanford Graduate School of Education and Marily Oppezzo, a Stanford PhD graduate in educational psychology, creative thinking increases both during and immediately after walking.

The research discovered that both indoor and outdoor walking stimulated creative ideas. The primary influence was the act of walking itself, not the surroundings. Creativity levels were consistently and considerably greater for individuals who were walking compared to those who were sitting across the board.

Many individuals anecdotally assert that they think best when walking. We may now be making progress in understanding why, according to Oppezzo and Schwartz, who published their findings in this week's issue of the Journal of Experimental Psychology: Learning, Memory, and Cognition.

Now let's discuss further about creativity, and the impact of walking on creativity.

The ability to develop or recognize ideas, alternatives, or possibilities that may be useful in solving issues, interacting with others, or entertaining ourselves and others is what we mean whenwe talk about creativity. To be creative, you need to be able to examine things in new ways or from a different viewpoint. This is aprerequisite for creative thinking. You must be capable of producing new possibilities or new options, among other things, in Personality traits associated with creativity

- People who are creative have a tremendous degree of energy, but they are also frequently quiet and at rest.

- People who are creative are typically intelligent, yet at the same time, they can be quite naive.

- People who are creative have a balance of irresponsibility and playfulness, often known as responsibility and lack of responsibility.

- Individuals who are creative move back and forth between a rooted sense of reality and their imagination and fantasy on either end of the spectrum.

- On the spectrum that runs from extraversion to introversion, creative people appear to have tendencies that are diametrically opposed to one another.

- Individuals who are creative often have a propensity toward androgyny and are able to overcome traditional gender role stereotyping on some level.

- The majority of people who are creative have a lot of enthusiasm for their job, but they also have the ability to be very objective about it.

- Because of their openness and sensitivity, creative people are frequently put in situations in which they are vulnerable to experiencing both a tremendous amount of misery and a large amount of pleasure.

Hippocrates, the father of medicine, is credited with writing that "walking is man's best medicine." This is undeniably true on a physiological level, and it also appears to be the most effective treatment for enhancing our creative capacities. This proverb of Hippocrates has been defended by great brains both in the past and in the present; the following are some of the names on that list: Nikola Tesla was known to take extended strolls through a city park on a daily basis and asserted that he developed his thoughts completely in his head during these walks before committing anything to paper. At Apple, Steve Jobs insisted on having "walking meetings" with business associates, particularly when creative issue-solving was required. Mark Zuckerberg and many other people in Silicon Valley today replicate this practice. Several well-known authors, such as Henry David Thoreau,

L.M. Montgomery, J.K. Rowling, and Ernest Hemingway have stated that walking is the only surefire approach to overcoming writer's block. Merlin Coverley created a book called "The Art of Wandering," which is 265 pages long and discusses how literary history has been impacted by bipedal travels. This is because so many writers have been enthusiastic walkers throughout history (Dean, 2020).

Experiments that were discussed in the chapter before this one reveal that people who exercise regularly have better memories throughout their entire lives. This is true even though exercise is beneficial. Why did these brilliant brains place such a high value on the simple act of walking? How exactly does it bring about brilliant creativity? Walking alone, as opposed to engaging in otherforms of exercise, has proven to deliver the best outcomes. The creative process can be stimulated, as established by scientific research, just by going for a walk. Walking was found to increase creative production by a factor of sixty percent, according to a study conducted at Stanford University. In the study, 176 individuals, most of whom were college students, were given a number of tasks that are typically used to test "divergent thinking," which is an essential component of highly creative cognition. For instance, in one of these activities, participants were tasked with listing many applications that could be made of a particular item. Responses were rated "novel" if the researchers determined that no other participant had thought of the proposal and that it was viable and realistic (Dean, 2020).

It is interesting to note that the results were the same whether the walking took place indoors (on a treadmill facing a blank wall) or outdoors (in a lovely area with plenty of natural beauty), which suggests that experiencing the natural environment while walking is not the inspiration trigger. Additionally, the creative boost lasted for a good few minutes after the walk was finished. Although the exact reason why this advantage occurs is not entirely understood, scientists do have a few hypotheses to explain it. It's possible that the fact that walking requires the simultaneous use of various sections of the brain is what makes the activity so effective at boosting creative thinking. In fact, the human brain is as enormous as it is, partly because walking while maintaining an upright position is such a difficult task. Simply coordinating our steps and keeping our balance when walking requires a significant contribution from a variety of different parts and regions of the brain. According to the findings of researcher Cathy Perlmutter, the dynamic interaction between the left and right hemispheres of the neocortex may be the key to understanding the motivational benefits of walking. In general, thinking that is logical and linear is connected with the left hemisphere of the brain, while creativity and intuition are associated with the right hemisphere of the brain, despite the fact that both sides of the brain are employed to some degree in any form of work. In addition, each hemisphere is responsible for governing an alternate side of the body: the left hemisphere is in charge of the right side of the body, while the right hemisphere is in charge of the left. It is possible that walking, which involves both the left and right sides of the body continuously as we move from one foot to the next with each step, enables better communication between the two hemispheres of the brain throughout the process of coordinating those motions.

Productivity

In a world loaded with consistent interruptions and requests, keeping up with concentration and productivity is fundamental to achieving success. Walking, a basic yet strong movement, can give you a jolt of energy and improve your capacity to think, bringing about expanded efficiency. By integrating standard walks into youreveryday practice and endeavoring to accomplish 10,000 steps a day, you can encounter improved focus, mental clarity, and increased efficiency. Walking stimulates the bloodstream and the conveyance of oxygen to the brain, working on mental capability. As you walk, your pulse increases and your blood vessels enlarge, taking into account a better course all through your body, including your mind. This expanded blood stream and oxygenation feed synapses, supporting ideal mental execution and assisting youwith keeping on track and alert. Taking some time off from work orday-to-day obligations to take a walk can lessen pressure, clear your brain, and allow you to return to your undertakings with a recharged center and a more useful outlook.

CHAPTER FOUR

Walking Improves CognitiveFunction

People have held the misconception for a very long time that when a task and walking are combined, both suffer. According to the findings of a study that was conducted at the Del Monte Institute for Neuroscience at the University of Rochester, this is not always the case. By altering the use of cerebral resources, some young people who are otherwise healthy are able to increase their cognitive function when walking. However, this does not imply that you should begin a challenging endeavor when you are still working off the cake that you consumed the night before.

In a recent study that was just published in Cerebral Cortex, Eleni Patelaki, a biomedical engineering Ph.D. student at the University of Rochester School of Medicine and Dentistry, together with her team, uncovered unexpected results about individuals' capacity to execute many tasks at the same time. When the researchers first began their work, they lacked any tools that would allow them to forecast how various people would fare in this area. Some of the participants were surprised to discover that it was simpler for them to execute numerous things simultaneously (also known as dual-tasking) than it was for them to perform each task on its own (also known as single-tasking). This conclusion was unexpected and noteworthy, given that the common thinking in the field implies that our performance typically declines in proportion to the number of tasks we attempt to juggle at the same time (*Walking Can Improve Cognitive Function*, 2022). As it relates to cognitive function, you stand to gain the following when you engage in walking the right way.

Walking increases cerebral blood flow

When performing more difficult tasks, the brain requires a greater supply of oxygen since it uses more energy. Even when we are at rest, the brain is responsible for approximately twenty percent of the body's overall energy consumption. This is because the brain is the organ that uses the most energy. Recent studies have proven that the heart is not the only organ responsible for supplying blood to the brain. Researchers came to the conclusion that when we walk, the force of our foot striking the ground causes a hydraulic wave to go upward through our blood vessels. This has the effect of dramatically altering and increasing the amount of blood that is supplied to the brain (Garcia et al., 2016).

Improved cognitive flexibility

Memory and cognitive ability have both been shown to improve with regular walking. Walking, as well as other forms of regular cardiovascular exercise, has been found to increase the size of the hippocampus, an area of the brain that is essential for the generation and maintenance of memories. Walking also increases the release of growth factors, which encourage the growth of new neurons and the building of connections between brain cells. These two processes are essential for memory enhancement and assist in its development. Walking on a consistent basis can improve cognitive flexibility, which is the brain's capacity to switch between different activities and think creatively. Cognitive flexibility is distinct from multitasking abilities in that it relates to the brain's ability to move between different tasks and think creatively. The prefrontal cortex, a part of the brain linked with executive skills such as problem-solving, decision-making, and creative thinking, is stimulated to produce new neurons when a person walks. Walking can help improve your cognitive flexibility, which in turn can help you conceive of new ways to solve problems and stimulate inventive thinking. Walking can be an effective way to lower levels of stress, which in turn has a beneficial effect on cognitive function. Memory, concentration, and the ability to makedecisions can all suffer from the effects of prolonged exposure to stress. Your brain will be able to work at its highest potential and be better able to deal with cognitive obstacles if you engage in physical activity such as walking. This type of activity can reduce stress and increase cognitive resilience.

Aim for regular, moderately intense walks that raise your heart rate if you want to get the most out of the cognitive benefits of walking. Walk at varying speeds, try out new routes, or add in extra challenges like walking uphill or incorporating interval training into your normal walking practice. These are all great ways to add variety to your normal walking routine. It is vital to have a well-rounded approach to brain health, including a good diet, appropriate sleep, mental stimulation, and social interaction. Walking can be extremely beneficial for cognitive function andbrain health, but it is also important to maintain a well-rounded approach to brain health.

Why cognitive flexibility is important: When circumstances change as they should, it is your good mental agility that counts foryour success. If you face a challenge, for example, you don't get flustered but instead handle it and seek out various potential answers, which helps you succeed when circumstances change. To maintain your resilience in the face of strain, which in turn is essential for maintaining good mental health, you require cognitiveflexibility. If you have a high degree of cognitive flexibility, you willhave an easier time juggling your career and your schoolwork, and you will be able to transition between different projects and clients with ease if the requirements or the due dates alter. You don't havefeelings of being overwhelmed when faced with new obstacles, and you're able to grasp new ideas and abilities more quickly and with less effort. This is of utmost importance when you are required to adjust to new ways of working, whether it is with a new kind of software, a new process, or new legislation. Additionally, you are not easily distracted and instead focus your attention on completing the tasks at hand.

While walking will greatly help your cognitive flexibility, it is also important to make it wholesome by engaging yourself actively in:

Expose yourself to new ideas. Discovering new things and actively expanding your knowledge can have a significant influenceon your own development as a person, as well as your cognitive talents and entire outlook on life. Let's dig more into the idea of expanding your mind and thinking through taking in new information, embracing curiosity, engaging in experimenting, and taking risks that you know are manageable. The completion of one's official education is by no means required to mark the end of one's quest for knowledge. Learning new things on a consistent basis, whether it is a new language, a musical instrument, a cooking technique, or the nuances of a new technology, helps to keep your mind active and flexible. Learning throughout one's life helps to cultivate a mindset that is receptive to both development and change. Exploration and innovation both require a healthy dose of natural curiosity. When you actively seek out new experiences, you stimulate your curiosity, which in turn motivates you to question things, investigate unexplored territory, and question the established order. To acquire new knowledge, one must be able to adjust to novel circumstances. This helps to create an adaptable mindset, which in turn enables you to deal with change more effectively in a variety of domains of life. The more you put yourself in situations where you are forced to venture beyond your comfort zone, the more accustomed your body and mind will become to doing so. Learning always entails some degreeof uncertainty and danger since it necessitates exploration of uncharted areas. You will develop a sense of resilience and adaptability if you take on the challenge of learning something newwillingly and with an open mind. Your confidence will increase as you progress through the learning process and demonstrate that you are able to overcome initial problems and disappointments.

Participating in activities that require ongoing learning helps boost neuroplasticity, which refers to the brain's capacity to rearrange itself through the formation of new neural connections. This phenomenon is essential for preserving cognitive health and putting off the onset of cognitive decline associated with advancingage.

Work on your emotional intelligence. Emotional intelligenceis defined as the capacity to recognize one's own feelings as well as those of other people, to channel those feelings into productive endeavors, and to keep those feelings under control while doing so.If you have high emotional intelligence, not only will you be a useful member of the team right now, but you will continue to be so in the future as well. If you have the ability to empathize with other people, also known as putting yourself in their situations, then you will be better able to comprehend and take into account the points of view of other people. It is very easy to dismiss colleagues who appear to be a pain in the neck, but challengeyourself to identify the strengths, skills, and perspective they bring to the table. Remember that cognitive flexibility means being open to listening to and taking into account various viewpoints and approaches to doing things. Keeping an open mind and being inspired to think in new ways are both benefits of maintaining relationships with people who have contrasting worldviews.

Your brain also needs a break. On the other side, in order for your brain to function correctly, it needs downtime, so make sure you give yourself some time to just zone out. Such as on those days off that are built into your schedule and during the breaks that are built into your walk-out schedule. It is not necessary for you to exert an excessive amount of effort for the entirety of the walkout. In a somewhat perplexing twist, this may also help develop your cognitive flexibility. If you let your mind simply wander, you mightfind yourself coming up with original thoughts and fresh perspectives on existing concepts.

Limit your distractions: anything that will not help you get closer to accomplishing your objective during the walk should be cut off. Your schedule should only allow you a certain amount of free time. This highlights how important it is to have a period of time during your walk that is undistracted and concentrated in order to get the most out of it. This involves turning down the volume on your phone, turning off any notifications, and selecting a path or setting that is favorable to the accomplishment of your goal. Your thought process can be disrupted, and your cognitive flexibility can be hindered, when you have distractions. Walking while remaining focused and avoiding distractions may be a useful means of personal and professional growth.

Improved ability to understand and analyze

The act of walking boosts blood flow to the brain, which ensures that the brain receives more oxygen and nutrients, both of which are necessary for cognitive activities. When your brain is well nourished, it can more efficiently accomplish tasks like understanding, analyzing, and comprehending. Walking provides an excellent opportunity for introspection and reflection. It helps you break away from the rush and bustle of everyday life, allowing your brain the space it requires to digest information and connect ideas. This is especially useful for in-depth comprehension and analysis.

As we've seen, engaging in physical activity, and more specifically, walking, can improve cognitive ability and make it easier to achieve one's full potential. It has been discovered that walking increases the amount of oxygen that is delivered to the brain, puts the brain in a creative state, and allows us to access our subconscious thoughts. All of these benefits can be quite helpful for performing complicated cognitive activities. However, not all mechanisms are well known; therefore, further research is necessary. The cumulative effect of these factors is improved brain health. You can improve the clarity of your thoughts and your ability to concentrate by making walking a regular part of your routine.

CHAPTER FIVE

Moods and Thoughts

Depression, or depressive disorder, is a frequent mental disorder. It involves a persistently downcast attitude or loss of enjoyment or enthusiasm for activities. It differs from typical mood swings and thoughts about day-to-day existence. It can have an impact on all facets of life, including interactions with friends, family, and the local community. It may be the cause of or a symptom of issues at work and in the classroom. Any person can experience depression. It is more likely to occur in people who have experienced abuse, significant losses, or other stressful situations. Depression is more common in women than in men. According to the World Health Organization, an estimated 3.8% of the population experiences depression, including 5% of adults (4% among men and 6% amongwomen) and 5.7% of adults older than 60 years. Approximately 280 million people in the world have depression (1). Depression is about 50% more common among women than among men. Worldwide, more than 10% of pregnant women and women who have just given birth experience depression (2). More than 700,000 people die by suicide every year. Suicide is the fourth leading cause of death in 15–29-year-olds (*Depressive Disorder (Depression)*, 2023).

How we feel can change how we see and enjoy life. The World Health Organization's report mentioned above should make us worried, especially if we're dealing with tough times. The report is concerning because people who are really sad often think about hurting themselves. So, what causes our moods to change? Well, studies have found that our mood is mostly controlled by tiny chemicals in our brain called neurotransmitters. These chemicals react to what's happening around us. Things we go through every day make us think, and those thoughts make us feel certain ways. Dopamine and serotonin are tiny molecules called neurotransmitters, and their job is to send signals all over our bodies. They have a big effect on our emotions. When our brains release dopamine, it gives us a short burst of happiness. On the other hand, serotonin is quite similar to dopamine but provides a longer-lasting sense of joy and feels good. These two substances also act as hormones, which are special chemicals that help controlmany different things inside our bodies. They help with stuff like how we grow, how we use energy, how we feel, and even how we sleep!

Dopamine

Dopamine is like a messenger chemical in our brain and body. People call it the "pleasure hormone" because it shows up when wedo things that make us happy. This system is set up to give us a little prize when we do stuff to keep ourselves healthy, like eating, drinking, competing to survive, and having babies. This little burst of excitement can make us feel like we want to do more of that thing. But here's the catch: It's just a quick feeling of being rewarded. Our bodies start wanting that good feeling more and more. That's why stuff like eating cookies or having sugary drinks, which boost our dopamine levels, can be so hard to stop. Once our bodies get a taste of dopamine, they keep wanting it over and over again.

Serotonin

Serotonin is a chemical that works as a messenger in our bodies. It tells our body how to do important things and helps manage our feelings, memory, sleep, body temperature, and hunger. Most of this serotonin is made in our stomachs, but some also comes from our brains. When your body has the right amount of serotonin, you might feel focused, happy, or peaceful. But when the levels are too low, it can affect your mood, sleep, and stomach. If your child needs more serotonin, you can help by having them go outside for a walk, get some sunshine, chat with friends or family, or eat foods that have something called tryptophan. Tryptophan helps our bodies make serotonin, and you can find it in things like milk, oats, cheese, and nuts. Studies show that people suffering from depression typically have decreased levels of serotonin and higher levels of cortisol.

If you frequently encounter stressful circumstances, your body experiences heightened stress hormone levels, subjecting it to substantial pressure. Similarly, if you lack a strong support system, you may have reduced levels of neurotransmitters, which are natural mood enhancers. Engaging in physical activity is recognized for its ability to mitigate the impact of stress and harmonize the brain's chemical composition, leading to an enhancement in emotional well-being. Conversely, an inequity in neurotransmitter levels can contribute to the development of depression. Two such neurotransmitters, serotonin and dopamine, both of which are stimulated through exercise, play pivotal roles in this regard. By consistently participating in a fitness regimen, such as regular walking, you can experience an improvement in your mood. Exercise like walking can be an effective treatment for mild to moderate mental health disorders without the need for medications and their side effects. Exercise can also be used as a complement to medication and therapy for moderate-to-severe mental health disorders. Other important mental health benefits include improved energy, lower stress levels, better sleep, increased mental clarity, improved social health and relationships, and improved self-esteem.

However, it's essential to understand that while walking can be beneficial, it may not be a standalone solution for everyone struggling with depression. Depression is a complex and multifaceted condition with various underlying causes, including genetic factors, brain chemistry imbalances, trauma, and life circumstances. These factors often necessitate professional intervention. Seeking help from a specialist, such as a psychiatrist or therapist, is crucial for several reasons. Firstly, they can provide a comprehensive assessment to determine the root causes of your depression and tailor a treatment plan accordingly. This may involve therapy, medication, lifestyle changes, or a combination of these approaches. Secondly, specialists can monitor your progress and make necessary adjustments to your treatment plan. Depression is not a one-size-fits-all condition, and what works for one person may not work for another. Specialists can adapt your treatment to ensure it remains effective. Moreover, they offer invaluable emotional support and guidance throughout your journey to recovery. Depression can be isolating, and having atrained professional to talk to can make a significant difference.

Walking helps deal with ruminating thoughts

Rumination is defined as the habitual recurrence of thoughts, which frequently prevents people from having more productive and goal-oriented thinking. Excessive and bothersome thoughts regarding unpleasant events and emotions are referred to as ruminating thoughts. Rumination is defined by the American Psychological Association as obsessional thinking, which involves agreat deal of recurrent thoughts that interfere with other types of thinking. It's as if you're caught in a mental hamster wheel and unable to escape the vicious circle of negativity.

Our brains have a tendency to get tied up in a variety of thinking patterns, which can make it difficult to determine whether we are engaged in problem-solving and self-reflection or whether we are simply repeating the same cycle of thought. If we have a greater understanding of the differences between these different types of ruminative thinking, we will be able to better manage our mental health and build more tailored techniques for coping. Rumination is a troublesome mental trap when we repeatedly replay self- perpetuating ideas or themes in our minds. Repetitive negative thinking frequently causes it as a result of:

- Tough experiences from the past

- Depression

- Anxiety

- Perfectionism

- Relationship worries

Why, though, is this cycle so bad for us? The truth is that ruminating and obsessive thinking can negatively affect our well- being, exacerbate any existing anxiety or sadness, change our eating patterns, and make it difficult for us to carry out daily tasks. In order to combat rumination and establish detached mental space from our thoughts, it is crucial to comprehend its causes and effects.

There is a growing body of evidence that suggests physical inactivity has replaced smoking as the new 'nicotine'. In other words, inactivity has become an epidemic at an epidemiological level. Studies have shown that high inactivity scores lead to higher early mortality rates as well as significant economic costs for individuals and public authorities (Dingle et al., 2016). Many mental health conditions, such as depression, anxiety, and phobias, as well as PTSD, can be triggered by ruminating thoughts. In some cases, however, rumination may simply be triggered by a specific traumatic event (e.g., a failed relationship). Long-term rumination can worsen the symptoms of already existing mental health conditions; however, being able to manage ruminating thoughts can help to alleviate these symptoms and promote relaxation and joy.

In a study, 129 inpatients, with a mean age of 38.16 years and 50.4% of them being female, participated in the study and filled out a questionnaire both immediately before and immediately after engaging in physical activity. Another round of questions was filled out by thirty other inpatients throughout the same week. Thequestionnaire included questions about socio-demographic factors as well as health-related topics. In addition, the questionnaire inquired about the respondent's current psychological states, including mood, rumination, social contacts, attentiveness, weariness, and physical strengths as a proxy for the respondent's physiological conditions.

The most important takeaways from the study were that inpatientswith mental problems who participated in the study reported increases in their mood, physical strength, concentration, and appreciation of social contact after participating in a single bout of exercise. At the same time, I noticed a reduction in rumination and exhaustion. In addition, the pattern of findings that were discusseddid move in a positive direction over the course of two sessions, which suggests that there is consistency in the changes that occur as a result of single bouts of exercise. The recent findings make an important contribution to the existing body of research bydemonstrating that inpatients with mental problems might show a minor but significant improvement in psychological aspects at the microlevel, which is to say, after only one session of exercise (Brand et al., 2018).

Anxiety and ruminating are two different mental processes that are related to one another. The mental process of dwelling on the past, known as rumination, can frequently make symptoms of depression and anxiety disorders much more severe. On the other hand, anxiety is characterized by an abnormally high level of worryand unease about the unpredictability of the future, both of which can lead to rumination. Being aware of the distinctions between ruminating and the symptoms of anxiety can assist one in better comprehending the individual implications that each has on our mental health and in the development of more effective coping techniques.

CHAPTER SIX

Stress Reduction

In today's tech-driven world, speed reigns supreme. Technology has turbocharged our lives, enabling lightning-fastaccomplishments. Yet, as progress accelerates, so do the challenges we face. We're expected to tackle life's complexities at the same rapid pace, often leaving us overwhelmed and anxious when we can't keep up. Stress becomes an unwelcome companion as we grapple with the breakneck speed of modern life. It seems as though stress is becoming an inseparable friend. It is a phenomenon that is shared by all people, a raging tempest that can rage within anyone, regardless of age, gender, or family history. Stress has two sides: one that can occasionally act as a motivator but also has a darker side, one that can have deep and lasting repercussions on the physical, mental, and emotional well-being ofan individual. One way to describe stress is as a state of worry or mental tension that is brought on by a challenging circumstance. The human body's normal reaction to adversity and danger is stress, which motivates us to find solutions to these problems. The way in which we react to stressful situations, on the other hand, has a significant impact on our health in general. Both the mind and the body can be affected by stress. A healthy dose of stress can be beneficial and make it easier for us to carry out our daily responsibilities. Problems with one's physical and mental health might be brought on by excessive stress. The ability to deal with stress in healthy ways is beneficial to our mental and physical health and can help us feel less overwhelmed.

A "fight or flight" reaction is activated in response to stress, which prepares you to either confront the source of the stress or flee from it. There are some situations in which stress might be beneficial. When it helps you escape an accident, for example, achieve a tight deadline, or have your wits about you in the midst of chaos, it can be beneficial to your health. There are times when we all feel anxious, but the things that stress one person out may be very different from the things that stress another person out. A thrilling experience such as skydiving would be a good illustration of this point. Some people thrive on the excitement it brings, while others can't even fathom the possibility of it happening. For example, the anxiety you feel before your wedding day can be considered a healthy sort of stress. However, stress should only be short-term. When you have successfully navigated the "fight or flight" moment, your respiration and pulse rate should both settle down, and your muscles should become relaxed. Within a short period of time, your body should revert to its natural state without experiencing any adverse consequences that will be permanent. On the other hand, excessive stress that occurs frequently or over an extended period of time can be damaging to both the mind and the body. It also happens rather frequently. Eighty percent of Americans who were polled said that they had experienced at least one sign of stress within the previous month. Twenty percent of those surveyed reported feeling under a high amount of stress. Due to the nature of life, it is not feasible to totally rid one's life of stress. However, we have the ability to learn to avoid stress whenever possible and to cope with it whenever it cannot be avoided.

Types of stressAcute stress

Everyone, at some point, experiences acute stress. It is the instant response of the body to a novel and difficult scenario. It's the kind of anxiousness you may experience after squeezing out of a car accident by a hair's breadth. It is also possible for it to originate from something that you really enjoy doing. It's the feeling you get when you're on a roller coaster or skiing down a steep mountain slope that's equal parts terrifying and exhilarating at the same time. These brief bouts of acute stress often won't cause any lastingdamage to you. Your health may even benefit from these experiences. Your body and brain get valuable practice in creating the optimum response to future stressful events when they are put through stressful conditions. When the threat is no longer present, your body's systems should go back to functioning normally.

Episodic acute stress

A condition known as episodic acute stress is one in which an individual endures a number of separate instances of acute stress. This is something that can happen if you tend to get scared and worried about things that you believe have a chance of happening. It may appear as though your life is in complete disarray and that you are always moving from one catastrophe to the next. A lot of professions, such as being a police officer or firefighter, can put you in high-stress circumstances on a regular basis. Occasional intense stress can be detrimental to both your physical and emotional health and well-being.

Chronic stress

This form of stress manifests itself over a protracted period of timeand is more detrimental. Examples of situations that might produce chronic stress include persistent poverty, the presence of dysfunction in the family, and marital dissatisfaction. It takes place when an individual is unable to perceive any way to avoid their stressors and ceases looking for answers to their problems. A stressful event that happens when a person is young could also bea cause of long-term stress. Chronic stress makes it hard for the body to get back to a normal level of stress hormone activity. This can cause problems with the heart, lungs, immune system, sleep system, and reproductive system.

A constant state of worry can also make it more likely for a person to get type 2 diabetes, high blood pressure, or heart disease. When stress is constantly present in a person's life, it can lead to the development of mental health conditions such as anxiety, depression, and PTSD (posttraumatic stress disorder). People can become accustomed to feeling anxious and despondent, which can allow chronic stress to continue without being recognized. It is possible for it to become ingrained in an individual's nature, rendering them perpetually vulnerable to the effects of stress, regardless of the circumstances in which they find themselves. People who suffer from chronic stress are at an increased risk of experiencing a mental breakdown, which may result in suicidal thoughts, acts of violence, a heart attack, or a stroke.

What causes stress?

When confronted with stressful circumstances, individuals respond in a variety of ways. It is possible that an experience thatis stressful for one person will not be stressful for another person, but the fact remains that practically any event has the potential to be stressful. Simply considering a trigger, or even multiple smaller triggers, can be enough to set off an anxiety response in some people. When confronted with the same source of stress, there is no discernible reason why one person might experience lower levels of stress than another. Some people's mental health concerns, such as depression or a growing sense of annoyance, injustice, and anxiety, can make it easier for them to feel stressed than others. The way a person responds to various sources of stressmay be influenced by their history. Among the common causes of stress observed are: lack of a job, job problems, lack of time or money for retirement, bereavement, family troubles, health issues, moving, marriage, divorce, abortion, or the loss of a baby, driving in heavy traffic or being afraid of an accident, fear of crime or problems with neighbors, pregnancy and becoming a parent, too much noise, pollution, crowding, and not knowing what will happen or waiting for something important. Just about anything can cause stress, depending on who is involved in the situation.

Managing stress

Long-term exposure to stress can be hazardous to various systems in the body and can even lead to health problems such as high blood pressure and a weakened immune system, in addition to mental diseases such as anxiety and depression, as explained earlier. When you are under pressure, not only does your body experience an increase in the "fight or flight" hormone adrenaline, but it also produces an increased amount of the stress hormone cortisol. This is essentially the chemical opposite of the hormone melatonin, which helps people fall asleep and stay asleep. Because of this, cortisol sends a signal to your body that now is not the appropriate moment to relax and digest, as there are other elements that require attention. Your capacity to concentrate, do many tasks at once, and control your emotions can be negatively impacted by elevated cortisol levels, which, over time, can play a role in the development of an elevated level of stress that is damaging to the body's systems.

According to a 2022 Stress in America survey by The Harris Poll on behalf of the American Psychological Association, on a scale from 1 to 10, where 1 means you have "little or no stress" and 10 means you have "a great deal of stress," the average reported level of stress for the previous month among all individuals was 5.0, andthis number has been relatively stable throughout the year 2020. However, in comparison to pre-pandemic levels (2021: 5.0, 2020:

5.0, 2019: 4.9, 2018: 4.9, 2017: 4.8, and 2016: 4.8), this level is

significantly higher. What's more, an alarming percentage of people said that stress influences their day-to-day functioning, and more than a quarter (27%) of those adults said that on most days, they are so stressed that they are unable to operate as a result of the stress. A little less than half of those under the age of 35 (46%) and more than half of black people under the age of 35 (56%) agreed with this statement. While each generation has its tension instigators, it does seem like this is a particularly tough time for Americans' mental health (*The Best Walking Plan to Help You Reduce Stress*, 2023).

It is common knowledge that regular exercise is beneficial to the health of all parts of the body. According to numerous studies, engaging in regular physical activity can enhance cardiovascular health, strengthen bones and muscles, and even lower one's risk of developing certain cancers. However, were you aware that workingup a sweat can help make the brain stronger? An increasing body of evidence suggests that being physically fit is one method to improve brain health and that maintaining a consistent exercise regimen might lessen the negative effects of stress on the body. It might not make sense at first, but even though exercise is a sort of physical stress, it can also help the body better manage other types of stress. On the other hand, if the stress is of the proper kind, it might actually make the body more resilient. According to studies, people experience lower levels of stress hormones like cortisol and epinephrine following bouts of physical activity. This is despite the fact that exercise initially causes an increase in the body's stress response.

From a physiological standpoint, it appears that physical activity provides the body with an opportunity to practice coping with stress. It compels the body's physiological systems, all of which are engaged in the stress response, to communicate with one another in a manner that is significantly closer than is typical. Communication occurs between the cardiovascular, renal, and muscle systems. The cardiovascular system also communicates with the renal system. Both the central nervous system and the sympathetic nervous system are responsible for all of these functions, and they are also required to communicate with one another. The real benefit of exercise lies in the fact that it trains the body's communication system. As our lifestyles become more sedentary, our bodies become less effective at responding to stress.

Although walking of any kind has several health benefits, one study discovered that a one-hour walk in natural surroundings considerably reduces stress because of the favorable reactions our brains have to it. In addition, spending time outside allows your body to produce vitamin D from the sun, which can assist in the treatment of seasonal affective disorder (SAD), more commonly referred to as winter depression. During the autumn and winter months, when it becomes dark so early, it is especially important to expose oneself to sunshine in the morning or in the middle of the day. The stress hormone cortisol can be dramatically reduced with as little as a 20- or 30-minute walk during your lunch break (Rogers,bcbsnc:bio/michelle-rogers, 2022).

CHAPTER SEVEN

Better Sleep

Sleep is an essential part of our bodies' natural processes, and it plays an important part in ensuring our overall health and well- being. It is not simply a state of dormancy; the body goes through its natural process of resting both the body and the brain when it sleeps. The act of sleeping may appear to be very easy at first glance. Getting comfortable, shutting your eyes, and allowing yourself to drift off to sleep is all that is required for the vastmajority of people. However, despite how straightforward it may appear, sleep is actually one of the most complicated and baffling bodily processes that science is aware of. If you are not getting enough sleep or if the quality of the sleep that you are getting is poor, you will probably be able to tell merely by how you feel. If you don't get enough quality sleep, your body and brain won't be able to function as effectively as they should. In addition, there is an entire subspecialty of medicine devoted solely to the study of sleep and the treatment of diseases that interfere with or impact it.

An exciting new study of lifestyle and sleep habits found that taking more steps during the day may be associated with better sleep at night. This was stated in an article written by Gretchen Reynolds and published in the New York Times on October 30, 2019. According to the findings of the research project that investigated the connections between walking and dozing off, simply being active can have an effect on how well we sleep, regardless of whether or not we actively engage in physical activity.Why are we concerned about sleep? It is a natural phenomenon, you may say, because everyone sleeps. New findings have shown that a large percentage of the adult population does not get as much sleep as they should.

Why sleep is important

Why is it critical to get sufficient sleep? If you don't get sufficient sleep, the world around you will start to feel like a terrifying dream. Things that appear to be of no consequence throughout theday become hideous. Worse of all, you are aware that if you go without sleep, you will be less prepared to find solutions to those problems when the sun rises. However, you do not stand alone. Every night, insomnia (sleeplessness caused by stress, disease, etc.) affects 70 million people in the United States. Poor sleephabits have repercussions for us not only at work but also in our personal lives, our finances, and our physical well-being.

During your time spent sleeping, a number of important things take place, including the following:

Taking care of the brain: During the time that you are unconscious, your brain is busy rearranging and cataloging the knowledge that you have learned. Comparing this to the work of a librarian at the end of the day, which involves organizing and stacking books, It makes gaining access to what you learn and recall, as well as making use of those items, easier and more efficient.

Efforts are made to save energy and store it. Throughout the course of the day, the cells in your body draw on the reserves ofresources they have stored in order to carry out their functions. When you're asleep, your body uses fewer resources than it does when you're awake. This allows those cells to replenish their supplies and prepare themselves for the following day.

Recuperation and personal repair: Your body will have an easier time healing wounds and repairing damage that occurred while you were awake if you reduce the amount of activity you get. That is also why you will feel more weary and have a greater desire for rest when you are ill.

Make or break your career: What role does sleep play in your professional life? If you don't get enough sleep on a consistent basis, your focus, reaction time, memory, and ability to make decisions will all suffer. It destroys your interpersonal skills, which are one of the most important factors in determining your professional success. Lack of sleep can also be a factor in accidents. Sleep deprivation played a significant role in disasters like the explosion on the Challenger space shuttle, the Exxon Valdez oil spill, and the nuclear meltdown at Three Mile Island. In fact, when it comes to motor function, speech, memory, decision-making, and problem-solving, workers who are exhausted are comparable to employees who are drunk. It is estimated that fatigue is the cause of 100,000 car accidents each year. In addition, when we climb the corporate ladder, we take on more responsibilities, which in turn results in less time spent sleeping. On average, senior managers and CEOs receive 25 percent fewer hours of sleep each week.

The connection between walking and sleep quality

Gretchen Reynolds reported to the New York Times that in a new study, which was published recently in sleep health, researchers at Brandeis University in Waltham, Mass., and other institutions decided to investigate whether and how walking could be linked with sleep.

This study was a component of a larger initiative that aimed to motivate adults in the greater Boston area to engage in more physically active pursuits. For the purpose of this project, the researchers recruited 59 largely middle-aged men and women from Boston and the surrounding area who worked full-time jobs and were concerned that they did not have enough time for physical activity in their schedules. These participants were each given an activity monitor by the researchers, and in some instances, they were also given advice on how to increase the amount of time they spent walking despite having busy schedules. (One of the purposes of the study was to compare the effects on activities of monitoring just versus monitoring in addition to delivering advice and encouragement.)

The volunteers were asked to wear the monitors for a period of one month so that data could be collected on the total number of steps they took each day as well as the total number of minutes spent moving in any capacity This exercise consisted of lighter chores, such as cleaning the house. During the course of the study, the participants also filled out a number of questionnaires at the beginning as well as at the conclusion of the four-week period. The participants were asked to rate the quality of their sleep, including how long it took them to fall asleep, how often they woke up during the night, and how refreshed they felt when they woke up the next morning, as well as the quantity of their sleep, which was determined by the hours that they said they went to bed and when they said they got up.

In the current study, the researchers looked over the data for each of the 59 people, paying particular attention to the amount of activity the participants had logged and how well they had slept, in the hopes of identifying detectable patterns. That is correct. In fact, it was found that there was a strong and persistent connection between moving around and falling asleep. In essence, the number of steps that a person took over the course of a month was directly correlated with how well they felt like they slept during that time period. The same thing happened when the researchers considered the amount of time the participants had spent moving; the more time an individual spent moving over the month, the higher they assessed their overall quality of sleep.

Even when the researchers looked at each day individually, they found that the connections still held. On any given day, if a person had done more steps than was typical for them, they normally reported having a higher quality of sleep that night. (Because the majority of the participants had already been sleeping approximately eight hours a night prior to the start of the trial, there were not many significant impacts on sleep length.) According to Alycia Sullivan Bisson, a doctoral student in psychology at Brandeis who co-conducted the new study with her mentor, Margie Lachman, and others, "I think it's fair to say" that these results show that individuals who move more also sleep better. "I think it's fair to say" that people who move more also sleep better. She also notes that the level of physical exercise necessary to achieve the desired improvement in sleep was not particularly taxing. The group of 59 participants walked an averageof a little over three and a half miles each day, which results in an average daily step count of approximately 7,000. Greater mileage covered was associated with better sleep, but even the least active participants found that increasing their mileage slightly on some days led to improvements in their sleep quality later on.

Why does going for a walk have such a profound effect on one's ability to sleep? Although the researchers can't say for sure, they think it may have something to do with the impulses that aretransmitted to your brain when you walk. To begin, there is the mental component. It is a well-established fact that going for a walk can alleviate symptoms of worry and despair, improve your mood, and make you generally happier. It is undeniably simpler to get to sleep and remain asleep when one goes to bed with a clear head and a sense of contentment about one's day. In addition, walking on a consistent basis teaches your body when it is appropriate to be active and when it is time to calm down and rest. Walking causes an increase in body temperature, which the National Sleep Foundation claims sends a signal to your brain. This signal tells your brain to lower your body temperature later in the day, which helps you get a better night's sleep. According to this article on SleepFoundation.org, people who suffer from chronic insomnia who engage in aerobic activity of moderate intensity, such as walking, see a reduction in the amount of time it takes them to fall asleep and an increase in the amount of time they spend asleep when compared to a night when they do not exercise.

When would you recommend going for a walk if you're having trouble falling or staying asleep? It is best to give yourself at least two hours before you want to go to bed, but the exact amount of time needed to allow your body to return to a normal temperature will vary from person to person. Therefore, pay close attention to how both your body and mind react on days in which you engage in a greater amount of physical exercise.

Do you want to get more restful sleep each night? Get out and take a walk. Both your mind and body will be grateful to you, and you may find that you have more vitality and are better able to refresh yourself so that you may achieve your objectives.

CHAPTER EIGHT

Walking and Education

Studying and learning have traditionally taken place at desks, with students and academics surrounded by stacks of books and papers. On the other hand, as our knowledge of the human brain and the process of learning expands, so too does our approach to educational theory and practice. Learning while walking is one example of an innovative method that is rising in popularity. This approach is proving to be a game-changer for a significant number of students, whether it is through neatly structured written materials or audio materials.

The Walking Classroom is a program that is run by the Alliance for a Healthier Generation. Students participate in the program by walking briskly together for twenty minutes while listening to the same kid-friendly podcast that is downloaded on their WalkKit (an audio player) or by using the newly released mobile app. The walks last for a total of twenty minutes. Each episode of the podcast begins with a brief message about health literacy and features a character value that is interwoven throughout the story. The downloadable Teacher's Guide has a variety of lesson plans and quizzes that assist educators in conducting fruitful discussions and reviews of the audio content. The content of the podcasts, which is aligned with state requirements, is suitable for students in grades 3 through 8. The subjects covered in podcasts range from English language arts to social studies to science and beyond.

The program carried out two separate studies. They were conducted to investigate the effects of "The Walking Classroom" program. The first study looked at students' short-term and long- term memory retention, as well as their cognitive function and mood after participating in an activity. The second study looked at the influence of the program on student health literacy and levels of physical activity both before and after a school year in which Walking Classroom programming was implemented. A total of three hundred and nineteen (319) fourth- and fifth-grade pupils from four different public schools located within a single county in North Carolina participated in the research. This group was reflective of the overall grantee population that utilized the walking classroom. The percentage of students who were eligible for free or reduced lunch was an average of 81.25 percent (2 schools were at 99%), and the percentage of kids who were proficient in reading at the end of the grade ranged from 28 to 52 percent. During the course of four testing periods, the students participated in a battery of tests designed to evaluate their learning(via podcast quizzes), mood (by PANAS-10), cognitive performance (via 3-minute timed multiplication tests), and attitudes toward learning (via lunchtime focus groups). The testingwas conducted at four different times: in the beginning (one week before the podcasts), after participants walked while listening to podcasts, after participants sat while listening to podcasts, and oneweek after the podcasts were provided (to determine how wellparticipants retained the information). (*Research Confirms Students Learn More When Walking and Listening to theWalking Classroom Podcasts*, n.d.)

According to the findings of the studies:

Walking helps students learn more and remember what they have learned

According to their performance on the 10-question comprehensiontest on podcast content, students showed noticeably higher levelsof learning when walking while listening to podcasts than when sitting while listening to podcasts. This was true for both short- term and long-term retention.

The mood of students can be lifted by walking

When participants walked while listening to podcasts, all positive affect markers improved, while negative affect markers dropped when participants sat while listening to podcasts. In a similar vein, negative-affect indicators all decreased after walking, suggesting that the Walk, Listen, and Learn program has a considerable beneficial influence on student mood and attitudes toward learning.

Students benefit from the positive and empoweringeffects of the walking classroom

The students said that walking while learning gave them the feeling of being joyful, healthy, educated, smart, and thrilled. Students reported feelings of being robust, relaxed, invigorated, cheerful, and aware after participating in the walking and learning activities.

Numerous studies have found a correlation between physical activity and improved mental performance, which is further evidence that walking is an excellent form of exercise. When they get back to class, students are in a better mood, they are more focused, and they are more inclined to participate in post-walk conversations. Students have been shown to have improved information retention, classroom behavior, and engagement after The Walking Classroom has been implemented, as well as improved performance on standardized tests. Teachers have frequently reported this improvement in information retention.Inactive children and children with low academic success stand to profit the most from The Walking Classroom's increased exercise and educational content. However, all students benefit from the increased activity and educational material. Teachers and professionals working with children outside of school hours have access to an innovative tool thanks to The Walking Classroom that helps them fulfill the needs of their pupils who have alternative learning styles such as attention deficit hyperactivity disorder (ADHD), dyslexia, or autism, the study added.

This surprising conclusion will not be unconnected with the fact that it has already been shown that when we walk, the heart pumps more oxygenated blood to the brain as well as the other tissues in the body. Recent studies have proven that the heart is not the only organ responsible for supplying blood to the brain. The researchers came to the conclusion that when we walk, the force of our foot striking the ground causes a hydraulic wave to go upward through our blood vessels. This has the effect of dramatically altering and increasing the amount of blood that is supplied to the brain. During either a period of rest or continuous walking at a speed of one meter per second, a small study consisting of 12 young adults was conducted and presented at the annual meeting of the Experimental Biology Society. Using ultrasound measurements of blood velocity waves and arterial diameters, the researchers were able to determine the cerebral blood flow rates to both sides of the brain. They discovered that although walking at a normal pace generates a smaller pressure wave than running does, walking at a normal pace improves blood flow to the brain even more than running does. Walking has been shown to improve divergent thinking and generate new ideas, both of which are beneficial to creativity. Walking is not likely to be effective for tackling highly focused problems such as calculating a mathematical solution, but after walking, individuals may be able to focus better on other things after recharging their energy reserves. (*The Benefits of Walking for the Brain and More | Walkolution,* 2022)

CHAPTER NINE

Enhances a Sense of Achievement

Albert Bandura, Ph.D., a psychologist at Stanford University, is credited with being the first to establish the concept of self-efficacyin 1977. A person's level of self-efficacy can be defined as their levelof confidence in their own abilities to successfully carry out a specific behavior. For instance, if you are certain that you can walk one mile without encountering any difficulties, then you have a high level of self-efficacy for the behavior in question. Your self- efficacy for walking a mile is low; on the other hand, if you are absolutely convinced that you would feel weary and need to stop after only a few feet of walking, then you have a low level of confidence in your ability to do so (Pekmezi et al., n.d.).

How does self-efficacy apply to health and physical activity?

According to the self-efficacy idea, if you have confidence in your ability to carry out a certain behavior successfully, you will have a greater propensity to engage in that behavior. For instance, if you believe that you can ski down a mountain without falling, you could be more likely to go down the hill than someone who thinks that engaging in such activities will result in bodily injury. This is because you have more faith in your own abilities. This idea has significant repercussions for the modification of health-related behaviors and has been implemented in a variety of health-related contexts, including diet, weight reduction, alcohol consumption, tobacco use, sun protection, and physical activity. According to a body of research, self-efficacy beliefs have an effect on whether or not new healthy behaviors are adopted, whether or not they are generalized to a variety of settings, and whether or not they are maintained over time. When it comes to adopting new behaviors, most people are reluctant to even give them a shot if they do not believe they are capable of carrying them out well. For instance, if a person has never played basketball before, he may be concerned about appearing inept in a pickup game and may be disinclined to give it an attempt. Similarly, a youngster may decline to try tennis if she is concerned that she will not be able to hit the ball over the net.

The extent to which health behaviors are able to generalize to new contexts is similarly influenced by self-efficacy, and this degree of generalization can change based on the activity, the environment, and even the time of year. For instance, a person may feel confident in his capacity to participate in certain forms of physical activity, such as walking, but not in his ability to participate in aerobics. In addition, the person might feel comfortable strollingdown a path with a companion but not in other settings (for instance, while they are walking alone on a treadmill). To make matters even more complicated, the person might believe they are able to walk regularly during the warm summer months, but they might be nervous about walking during the cold winter months because of the unpredictable weather. There is a strong correlation between having self-efficacy in one domain and having confidence in another domain. For instance, if you have already attained a high level of proficiency in ice skating, you might have a more positive outlook on your ability to pick up roller skating. Beliefs about one's own capacity to succeed play a part in one's ability to continue engaging in healthy behaviors throughout time. In fact, a recent study demonstrated that self-efficacy predicted themaintenance of physical activity among people 5 years after completing a 6-month walking program (McAuley et al. 2007). This was found in a group of individuals who had previously participated in the walking program. Because of the numerouspositive effects on one's health that may be achieved by leading an active lifestyle, this is a very significant problem. Clients frequently report feeling confident about beginning a program of physical exercise, but they then voice concerns over their capacity to chooseto remain active on a continuous basis throughout the course of a longer period of time. After the first phase of excitement has passed, what is required to turn physical exercise into a habit is a wide variety of tactics as well as perseverance in the face of challenges.

How to develop self-efficacy

According to Bandura's theory of self-efficacy, there are four primary sources of influence that contribute to the growth of one's own sense of self-efficacy: one's own prior performance, vicarious experiences (such as watching others perform), verbal persuasion, and physiological clues. It is generally agreed that looking at one's previous successes is the most effective way to build self-efficacy (Pekmezi et al., n.d.). When a person sets a goal of walking one mile, for example, that sense of achievement exudes confidence to take on the next activity, and here is where walking comes in. A positive habit, such as going to the gym regularly, is formed by the gradual accumulation of positive behaviors over time. When you walk the same path every day without fail, you open the door to a plethora of benefits that go well beyond the act of walking itself.

Increasing One's Self-Confidence: The simple act of completing your walking route, whether it be a daily stroll through the neighborhood or a weekly journey through nature trails, makesa substantial contribution to the development of one's sense of self-confidence. You are reiterating your dedication to achieving a goal, even if it is a straightforward one, whenever you successfully complete one of your predetermined walks. This pattern of behavior inculcates a sense of accomplishment in you and serves as a gentle reminder that you are able to establish and attain goals.

Setting goals for oneself and achieving them, no matter how insignificant those objectives may seem, is an excellent way tobuild confidence. This newly discovered confidence does not stay confined to your walking habit; rather, it frequently spills over intoother aspects of your life. As you become more aware of your ability to overcome the obstacles along your walking route, you become more eager to face obstacles in your professional life, personal relationships, or pursuit of personal development.

A feeling of success and accomplishment: When you finish your walking path, whether it was a brisk 30-minute stroll or a multi-mile walk, you will feel a tangible sense of success. This is true regardless of the length of the walk. The sensation of having accomplished something is absolutely necessary for sustaining one's drive and keeping a positive outlook. When a goal is accomplished, the brain responds by releasing dopamine, achemical that is linked to feelings of pleasure and reward. Therefore, when you reach the end of your walk, your brain will reward you for this achievement, which will in turn keep you motivated to keep going. The use of this form of positive reinforcement can be an effective aid in the maintenance of a consistent walking program.

In addition, the feeling of success you get from walking might motivate you to create and achieve more substantial objectives in your life. It serves as a reminder that even the most arduous undertakings can be achieved with determination and constant work on the part of the individual.

Making Goals and Tasks More Attainable: The process of establishing and accomplishing goals while participating in a regular walking regimen can have a domino effect, making it easierfor you to achieve other goals in other areas of your life. This demonstrates how important it is to celebrate even the smallest victories. As you make progress towards the goals you set for yourself regarding your walking, you might find that you start to apply the same concepts to other aspects of your life. You may, for instance, use the self-discipline and determination that you've earned through walking to create clear, measurable goals at work and then apply those skills to attain those goals.

Walking on a consistent basis can also lead to improvements in your physical fitness, which, in turn, can have a positive impact on your general health and well-being. Because of your enhanced energy and stamina, you should find it easier and more expedient to complete the chores you face on a regular basis. Your ability to effectively complete your walking path can be viewed as a microcosm of your ability to successfully manage and complete your day-to-day tasks.

The Never-Ending Circle of Inspiration: The successful completion of your walking path will put you in a positive cycle of increased motivation. You acquire self-assurance and a sense of accomplishment with each walk, which motivates you to create new goals that are just a little bit more difficult. As you pass each of these new benchmarks, your self-assurance will increase, which will encourage you to venture into uncharted territory in your walking routine as well as in other aspects of your life. When it comes to achieving long-term objectives, this cycle may prove to be quite helpful. You can remind yourself that patience and constant effort are the keys to success by thinking back on your track record of finishing your walking route whenever you are confronted with a challenge that appears to be impossible to overcome.

CHAPTER TEN

Enhances Brain Health DuringAging

～✗

Our rapidly aging society faces a significant challenge in the formof dementia. In addition to lowering the standard of living of those who are afflicted, it also has a negative impact on patients' immediate families, forcing spouses or children to take on the role of caregivers and frequently putting financial pressure on households. Most cases of dementia are caused by Alzheimer's disease (AD), although dementia with Lewy bodies, vascular disease, front temporal degeneration syndromes, and a variety of other less prevalent conditions also contribute. Mild cognitive impairment (MCI), which affects more than 10% of people over the age of 70 and more than 20% of people over the age of 80, is a condition that has less of a negative impact on quality of life than Alzheimer's disease but is still rather common. Mild cognitive impairment (MCI) is frequently a precursor to dementia (Ahlskog et al., n.d.).

According to the findings of a new study, taking just 4,000 steps every day can lower the risk of dementia by one quarter in people who are unable to walk as far as 10,000 steps per day can reduce the risk of dementia in people who can walk that far. According to the article that was published in JAMA Neurology, an analysis of data from more than 78,000 people found that a half-hour of walking at a fast pace was associated with a 62% drop in the risk of dementia. This information was derived from the analysis of the data.

According to the first author of the study, Borja del Pozo Cruz, whois an adjunct associate professor at Southern Denmark University and a senior researcher in health at the University of Cadiz in Cadiz, Spain, "probably the biggest takeaway is that 10,000 steps may be the optimal number of steps to reduce the risk of dementia,cutting it by 50%." It has been proven that "faster steps provide superior results."

Another analysis of the same data, which was published in JAMA Internal Medicine, discovered that participants who walked quickly, at a pace of around 80 to 100 steps per minute, even for short periods of time, had a 30% lower chance of having dementia compared to people who walked nearly the same amount but at a slower pace. This finding was published alongside the finding that people who walked the same amount but at a slower pace had a higher risk of developing dementia. In addition to this, they had a lower risk of acquiring cardiovascular disease and cancer. The findings indicated that even a moderate amount of physical activity, such as walking at a brisk pace for a few thousand steps, can have a positive impact on health outcomes. "Walking is associated with better vascular profiles, which is probably the clearest pathway through which steps may benefit dementia," PozoCruz said in an email. "Steps may be beneficial for dementia. Therefore, it is "likely that vascular dementia is most preventable through physical activity."

According to the Mayo Clinic, vascular dementia is defined as a form of dementia that is "caused by brain damage from impaired blood flow to the brain. " According to the Alzheimer's Society, it is the type of dementia that occurs most frequently following Alzheimer's disease. The third most prevalent form of dementia is vascular dementia. Four thousand (4000) steps per day is less intimidating than 10,000 for many, so it may be a powerful message to motivate the most inactive and less fit individuals," Pozo Cruz said (Walking This Number of Steps Every Day Can Reduce Dementia Risk by 50%, n.d.). While walking 10,000 steps cut the risk of dementia by half, the study showed that a smaller number of steps, around 4,000, could cut the risk by a quarter. Pozo Cruz and his colleagues looked at data from the United Kingdom Biobank, which has been collecting biological and medical information on half a million people who volunteered to join the databank when they were between the ages of 40 and 69 since 2006, to investigate the impact that walking has ondementia. The participants in the databank were between the ages of 40 and 69.

The period of time from February 2013 to December 2015 was the primary focus of the study. Participants who had previously taken part in the biobank were extended an invitation to take part in the new study. As a condition of their participation, they were obliged to keep an accelerometer on their wrists around the clock, seven days a week. Pozo Cruz and his colleagues focused their study on 78,430 participants aged 40 to 79 who were free of cardiovascular disease, cancer, and dementia at the beginning of the study and who had at least three days' worth of data from accelerometers. In October 2021, the researchers conducted a follow-up examination of the participants by looking at their medical records and death certificates.

Following the individuals for a median of 6.9 years, Pozo Cruz and his colleagues came to the conclusion that 866 of the original participants had developed dementia by the year 2021. The number of steps people took per day was connected with how likely they were to develop dementia, with 9,826 steps per day being associated with a 51% decrease in the risk of dementia. The researchers found that the number of steps people took per day was associated with how likely they were to develop dementia. When people moved with a "purposeful" stride, the highest decrease, 57%, was related to 6,315 steps per day, and a step count of 3,826 was connected with a 25% decrease in the risk of dementia. Walking at a pace of 112 steps per minute for 30 minutes was linked with a 68% drop in risk, which was a discovery that drew a lot of attention because it was associated with such a significant reduction in risk.

Because more of the Biobank individuals will have reached an age when dementia is more widespread, Pozo Cruz believes that the benefits linked with doing 10,000 steps may turn out to be even bigger than what the study has already found when there are more years of follow-up. In recent years, there has been "an important trend to focus on modifiable risk factors for dementia that we can adjust in our own lives that may be important for living long and well," according to Emily Rogalski, Ph.D., associate director of the Mesulam Center for Cognitive Neurology and Alzheimer's Disease at Northwestern University's Feinberg School of Medicine in Chicago. Rogalski is quoted as saying that the focus on these risk factors has been "an important trend."

"We've also seen how exercise interventions and lifestyle changes can modify the risk of dementia," said Rogalski, who was not involved in the current study. "We've seen how exercise interventions and lifestyle changes can modify the risk of dementia. "I believe that this research presents a significant opportunity to investigate how the number of steps that we take and the intensity of those steps may play a role in the risk of dementia as well as in the health of our brains," said Dr. David Healy, who led the study.

According to Rogalski, the new study investigates the topic in greater depth by focusing on the optimum number of steps as well as the intensity of those steps. She went on to say that it is highly improbable that walking would turn out to be the only kind of exercise that affects the risk of dementia. "With interventions like exercise and cognitive stimulation, it's unlikely that there will be a one-size-fits all strategy," Rogalski said. "It's unlikely that there will be a one-size-fits all strategy. She went on to say that the most essential thing on an individual level is to combine scientific knowledge with what works best for that person (Walking This Number of Steps Every Day Can Reduce the Risk of Dementia by 50%, n.d.).

CHAPTER ELEVEN

Improved Heart Health and a Lower Risk of Stroke

Walking is one of the best exercises for maintaining a healthy heart because it gives you benefits with each step you take. According to the American Heart Association, it can enhance your cholesterol levels, blood pressure, and energy levels, and it can also help you combat weight gain, all of which contribute to an overall improvement in your heart health. Walking can also help you feel better about yourself by relieving stress, clearing your mind, and boosting your mood. What's the best part about the fact that doing all of those things can help minimize your risk of heart disease and stroke? You simply need around two and a half hours of moderate activity per week, like going for a brisk walk around the park.

If you have a profession that requires you to be sedentary for the majority of the day, it can be far simpler to just talk a good game than it is to actually walk the walk. It is possible to find pockets of time for cardiovascular fitness in the form of walking if you take the effort to study your daily routine and look for such pockets of time. Make use of the health advice included in this book under the supervision of your primary care physician.

When you've established a solid routine with walking and assume your body is up to it, you might want to think about adding some of these brief exercises to your regimen:

Walking Lunges: To perform a full lunge while walking, take a step that is significantly larger than your typical step and bring your back knee as close to the ground as you can. Step forward with the back foot in the same manner, and then step forward with the front foot. Repeat the lunges for a total of ten reps each time, if at all possible.

Walking curl press: Bring a pair of light weights with you, preferably dumbbells that weigh no more than three pounds, so that you may perform walking curl presses. Beginning with the weights in each hand down by your thighs, walk in this starting position. Curl the weights up to your shoulders, and then push them overhead. Bring the weights up to your shoulders in a curl. Bring the weights back down to your shoulders, and then bring them all the way back to your thighs. If at all possible, repeat the process in increments of three minutes.

Perform the Knee-Tap March: walk forward with your knees slightly bent and tap your hands on your knees after each stride. If at all possible, repeat the process in increments of three minutes.

You will likely be able to increase the number of aerobic and resistance workouts you perform once you have some patience, put in some practice, and remain persistent. And while the rule of two and a half hours of exercise each week is a fantastic starting point, it is possible that additional physical activity will be beneficial if you have the opportunity to do so. According to the CDC, seven hours of weekly physical activity could cut the risk of premature death by as much as 40 percent when compared to less than thirty minutes of action on a weekly basis. If you want to enhance your heart health, you shouldn't let excuses stop you from focusing on how to do it. Just get out there and walk. It doesn't matter if you call it a jaunt, a stroll, a saunter, a trek, or a promenade. Your coronary system will be grateful to you.

After having a stroke, increasing the amount that you move can be a huge help to your recovery as well as your self-confidence and overall health. Additionally, it can assist you in maintaining your health after having a stroke. Getting moving again after a stroke is likely one of your top priorities, but once your rehabilitation is through and you've been discharged from the hospital, how can you keep up the good work? Begin slowly and steadily increase your pace; don't try to accomplish too much all at once. Because of this, it is important that you figure out what works best for you because everyone is different. You may gradually include moreactivity into your everyday routine, whether you're at home or at work. You can find new ways to keep active regardless of whether you are standing, sitting, by yourself, or with others. (*Getting Moving After a Stroke*, 2019)

If you are concerned about your health after having a stroke and staying active, you can consult the chapter in this book that is devoted to frequently asked questions (FAQs) or talk to a member of the medical staff about the type of exercise that is most suitable for you.

CHAPTER TWELVE

You Get Fresh Oxygen and Sunlight (outdoor walking)

Many people have the experience of being imprisoned by their busy schedules, as they are unable to get out into nature as frequently as they would like. In addition, having a hectic schedule at home makes it difficult to sneak away from the house every once in a while. On the other hand, research has shown that maintaining a healthy brain can be helped by going for a daily walk outside. It is well worth your time to go for a stroll, even if all you have is ten minutes to spare. Take a look at this list of the four ways that your brain will benefit from going for a walk outside in the fresh air. Many positive effects on one's health can be attributed to breathing in fresh air. Today is a sunny day, and with sunrises occurring so early in the morning and sunsets occurring so late in the evening, there is no better time than the summer to get outside and take in some healthy doses of oxygen. A steady supply of new oxygen is required for every cell in your body, and as a result, every function that your body performs depends on oxygen. If you spend a significant amount of time indoors or in a place that is air conditioned, you may end up breathing the same air over and over again, which can make the air feel stuffy and stale. The simple act of going outside and taking in some oxygen- rich air can confer a significant number of positive effects on one's health.

Fresh air helps your brain and clears your lungs

This idiom is one that you have probably encountered at some point in your life. It is said that going outside and getting some fresh air can make a person feel better. However, not a lot of people are aware of the positive effects that being outside can have on the brain. Oxygen is vitally necessary for the proper functioning of a healthy brain as well as for its growth and recovery. In fact, healthy neuronal function in the brain requires approximately three times the amount of oxygen that is required for good muscular function. The brain is quite sensitive to changes in the amount of oxygen that it receives. Therefore, going for a walk outside and getting some fresh air might really increase a person's brain function. This is especially true for people who spend the majority of their day locked up in an office. Especially in enclosed spaces that have insufficient ventilation, the ratio of oxygen, nitrogen, and carbon dioxide in the air within is frequently not as healthy as it may be. Even if keeping plants indoors can be of assistance, there is no substitute for going outside to breathe in some fresh air. Outdoor air often contains higher concentrations of oxygen (not to mention lower levels of pollution) compared to the air found inside buildings. Your blood vessels in your lungs will dilate when you are exposed to more oxygen, which will improve the cleaning and tissue repair processes within your lungs as well as make it easier for your lungs to exchange gases. In a single action, you not only clear up your lungs but also assist your body in getting rid of items it does not require.

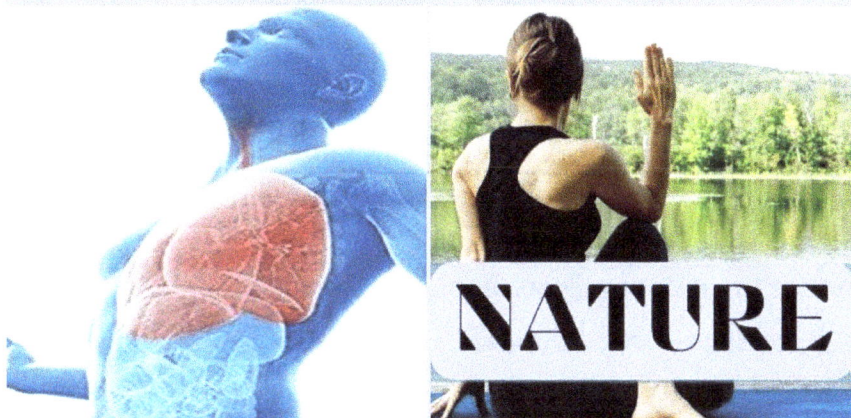

FRESH AIR HELPS THE BRAIN

A higher level of vitamin D

A person's skin is able to produce vitamin D, which is a vital mineral for maintaining good brain function, when exposed to sunlight. The inflammation in the brain is also reduced by vitamin D, which also helps to protect the neurons there. Vitamin D has also been linked to the manufacture of neurotransmitters and the proliferation of nerves, which has led researchers to make these correlations. Since all of these are necessary for our day-to-day functioning, vitamin D is of utmost importance. Despite this, vitamin D deficiency is becoming more prevalent with each passing year. You may get part of the vitamin D you need by going outside and exposing yourself to the sunlight. To reiterate, it is still beneficial for you to go outside, even if you can only do so for ten minutes.

It has the potential to boost your energy levels and mental concentration

The amount of oxygen in your blood will increase as a direct result of your lungs taking in more fresh air. If your blood contains a higher concentration of oxygen, then more of it will circulate to your brain. This will make you feel more energized, and it will also increase your capacity to concentrate and recall information. The Human Cognitive Neuroscience Unit in Northumbria conducted a study in which they found that volunteers who were given oxygen rather than ordinary air performed up to twenty percent better ona memory test. Additionally, it can help boost the creation of serotonin, which can result in a happier and less nervous state of mind for the user. All it takes is a few deep breaths of fresh air, andyour mind will become more organized, sharper, and more at ease (Kaplan, 2020).

Reduce the risk of airway bone infections

Taking deep breaths of clean air can help minimize the risk of contracting an airborne sickness or infection. This is due to the factthat germs like bacteria and viruses have a lower probability of surviving in clean air. When compared to the warm, humid, and indoor surroundings in which they thrive, there is a stark contrast.

It speeds up the healing process

The process of recovering from illness or injury may be quite stressful on the body. It seems logical that the repair or replacement of damaged cells would result in an increase in the amount of oxygen that your body requires. It has been demonstrated that oxygen therapy can increase recovery time for athletes, but simply going outside and getting some fresh air can also help you feel better and heal faster (Kaplan, 2020).

We may improve our well-being in a variety of ways, from feeling happier and more relaxed to having a measurable influence on our circulatory systems, recovery time, and overall health. Getting more fresh air and sunlight can help improve our well-being in a variety of ways. If you are feeling tense, exhausted, lethargic, or even plain bloated, you should walk outside and take some nice, deep breaths of fresh air.

CHAPTER THIRTEEN

Stimulates Brain Growth Factors

BDNF, which stands for brain-derived neurotrophic factor, is both a growth factor and a peptide (a type of long-chain protein). The word "nerve" derives from the Greek word "neuro," which also gives us the word "trophis," which means "pertaining to food, nourishment, or growth. In a nutshell, BDNF ensures the continued existence of neurons and other brain cells, encourages the formation of synaptic connections between neurons, and is necessary for the learning process as well as the storage of long- term memories. When it comes to adults, BDNF also plays an important role in the process of neurogenesis, which refers to the production of new neurons from stem cells. Although BDNF can be found in other parts of the body, such as the kidneys, blood plasma, and saliva, it is found in the brain and central nervous system, where it performs its most significant roles.

Walking isn't usually the first form of exercise that comes to mind when we think of activities that can improve our mood and make us healthier. The majority of us are aware of the advantages that running and other forms of high-intensity workouts have on raising endorphins, but neuroscientist Shane O'Mara believes that strolling could be just as beneficial to you. O'Mara, the author of the book "In Praise of Walking," recently gave an interview to the Guardian in which he asserted that walking might boost one's level of happiness as well as one's health and intellectual capacity. "Getting people to engage in physical activity before they engage in a creative act is very powerful," he says, but "getting people to move around before they create something is even more powerful. My theory, which we need to test, is that the activation that takes place throughout the entirety of the brain during problem-solving becomes significantly greater, almost as an accident of walking, demanding lots of neural resources," he added (How Increasing Your Walking Could Make You Happier and Better for Your Health, 2020).

It is common knowledge that physical activity has a beneficial influence on the human psyche. In his book, O. Mara says that walking stimulates the production of a substance called brain- derived neurotrophic factor (BDNF), which "may be thought of as a kind of molecular fertilizer created within the brain because it encourages structural remodeling and growth of synapses after learning... BDNF has been shown to boost resistance to the effects of aging as well as damage caused by trauma or infection. It is a common misperception, according to him, that walking does not qualify as actual exercise. He argues that people who go to the gym are typically more inactive for a longer period of time following their workout.

"This is a terrible mistake," he says. What we need to do is be significantly more generally active throughout the course of the day than we already are. If you have people wear activity trackers, you will notice that after they have participated in particularly strenuous activity for an hour, they engage in significantly less activity for the remaining hours of the day.

Walking and BDNF levels

According to a number of studies, the type of physical activity that is best suited to elevating your BDNF levels is strenuous aerobic exercise. Although there is an immediate increase in BDNF levels following exercise, it seems that the benefits are enhanced when exercise is performed on a consistent basis. High-intensity interval training (HIIT) may also be useful at increasing brain-derived neurotrophic factor (BDNF), according to a mini-review conductedin 2018, but the available data is quite limited. In addition, research conducted in 2017 found that resistance training can help increase BDNF levels in the body.

The researchers discovered that hypertrophy training (bodybuilding-style training) to the point of muscular fatigue elevated BDNF levels more than pure strength training does. However, if you are not already in the habit of exercising, increasing the amount that you move around may be one of the most effective strategies to raise your BDNF levels. Physically active adults, as opposed to sedentary people, have higher levels of the neurotrophic factor BDNF, according to a study published in Neuroscience in 2018.

How exactly can physical activity boost BDNF levels?

To this point, very few researchers have attempted to explain how exactly exercise increases the amount of BDNF that is circulating in the blood. BDNF may be released during exercise from the brain, skeletal muscle, peripheral blood mononuclear cells (PBMCs), vascular endothelial cells, and platelets, as suggested by a review that was published in 2018 and authored by Walsh et al. The authors hypothesize that the shear stress caused by the increased blood flow that occurs during exercise prompts many of these cells to release a greater quantity of BDNF from their storagethan they normally would.

CHAPTER FOURTEEN

Improved Blood Circulation

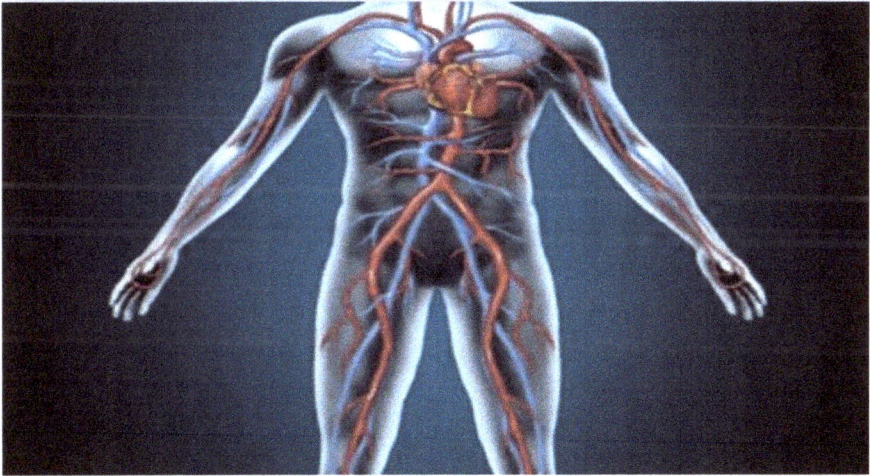

The movement of blood through our bodies, often known as circulation, is critical to maintaining good health. The delivery of oxygen to all parts of the body and its role in the elimination of waste are two of the many ways that healthy circulation benefits our many biological systems. Symptoms of poor circulation, in which the blood does not flow as vigorously as it could, can include tired or heavy legs, cold fingers and toes, low levels of energy, and even dull skin. Exercising regularly is one simple technique to improve one's circulation. You'll find that you have a bit more pep in your step once you get your heart racing; it's simply a matter of how much.

A well-circulated blood supply in the legs not only enables the tissues to take in nutrients and rid themselves of waste but also serves as a crucial function in the maintenance of long-term leg health and strength. Inadequate circulation in the legs can be improved by establishing some basic habits and making some dietary adjustments. The continuous movement of blood throughout the body, which is made possible by the pumping activity of the heart, is referred to as circulation. Blood is said to "flow" through the body because it moves via a network of tubes known as the circulatory system. Both arteries and veins are types of blood vessels; however, arteries are those that carry blood away from the heart, while veins are those that bring blood towards the heart. Because the blood needs to be pushed downward throughthe body in order to reach the heart from the lower sections of the body, the circulatory system must exert a great deal of effort in order to accomplish this task. When the muscles that surround the veins flex, they promote the flow of blood toward the heart, which in turn helps the circulation. Because of this, maintaining an activelifestyle, even if it's simply going around the block, can improve circulation. As we get older, our circulation could get worse. However, circulation issues can affect people of any age who are inactive for a significant portion of their day. Here are some useful pointers that will assist you in enhancing the blood circulation in both your legs and the rest of your body.

What Leads to Poor Circulation

Obesity, anemia, untreated blood clots, uncontrolled diabetes, and high blood pressure are just a few of the factors that can cause poor circulation. Smoking can also contribute to poor circulation. Peripheral artery disease is a condition in which restricted arteries decrease the flow of blood. The following are signs that may indicate that your circulation is not functioning properly:

- Insufficient amounts of energy or concentration

- Cold extremities (hands and feet)

- thinning of the hair or the loss of hair

- Healing that is either slowed down or delayed as a result of a weaker immune system

- Erectile dysfunction in men

Actions you should take

Walking is an easy, low-impact form of exercise that can assist you in developing a more physically active and healthy lifestyle, and it also has the potential to facilitate weight loss. Walking at any speed is excellent for increasing blood flow throughout the body since it is the best way to lower blood pressure and improve muscle contraction in the legs. Walking is also beneficial for increasing blood flow throughout the rest of the body. When the muscles in the legs contract and relax, they compress around the big veins in the legs, which helps to promote good circulation in areas where flow is more stagnant. To get your heart rate up and your blood flowing through your body, you don't have to be an Iron Man triathlete. In fact, any form of exercise that increases heart rate will improve your circulation. This involves going for walks. Even among those who have peripheral artery disease, which is a narrowing of the arteries that causes a reduction in circulation, even 20 to 30 minutes of brisk walking most days of the week has been demonstrated to enhance circulation. This is especially true for the legs. Walking for an extended period of time can, over time, help strengthen your heart and enhance your overall cardiovascular health. It is essential for one to have a functioning cardiovascular system in order to have good circulation.

Quit your bad habit: If you want your blood vessels to be healthy, then you should avoid smoking at all costs. In addition to increasing the risk of developing blood clots, smoking can cause swelling in the feet and ankles. If you smoke, your heart is not working in optimal conditions, and this can lead to damage in your blood vessels and veins in your legs.

If you quit smoking, your heart will be in better shape.

Position Your Body: When you sit on a chair, if you have a habit of crossing your legs, you may be impairing the circulation in your lower body. This popular position restricts circulation to the legs, making it more difficult for blood to reach the tissue in your legs and keep it healthy. Because of this, this position is not recommended. Make it a habit to sit in a position that is healthier for circulation, and try to maintain that position throughout the day.

You can improve your vein circulation by sitting in one of these positions, which are all recommended:

- Take a seat on the floor with your feet flat on the ground and your legs slightly separated from one another. Keep in mind that you need to rise up from time to time in order to avoid remaining in this position for an excessive amount of time.

- You can also try sitting with your legs slightly elevated to improve blood circulation. Put your feet up on a stool or ottoman that is raised anywhere from six to twelve inches off the ground.

- Increase the blood flow to your legs by propping them up on a pillow as you sleep. Additionally, your spine will thank you for adopting this position!

Stretching: Stretching on a daily basis is associated with a multitude of health benefits for the body. When done correctly, stretching can assist in improving blood circulation, which carries oxygen and nutrients to your organs and muscles, all of which are important for optimum function, movement, and flexibility. If you stretch with the correct technique, this benefit may be maximized.

CHAPTER FIFTEEN

Increased Focus and Attention

The ability of our brains to focus on one primary activity at a time has become more challenging to accomplish in today's rapidly advancing digital environment. You can, however, teach your mind to ignore distractions and stay in the here and now with the appropriate mentality and a little bit of effort. No matter how big or small the work at hand may be, having an awareness of the benefits of maintaining focus can be critical to your success. This awareness can also assist you in determining areas of your professional career in which you can make improvements. A person's ability to pay attention to, or concentrate on, a certain person or thing is referred to as focus. A person's attention is said to be focused when it is directed on a particular focal point. When it comes to their work, an employee is said to be focused when their attention is directed on the accomplishment of their primary aim or objective.

Regular exercise not only helps keep your brain refreshed, but it also stimulates it. Participating in physical activity will not only help you remember more but will also improve your general attentiveness. According to the findings of several studies that were referenced previously, not only will physical activity assist you in maintaining your energy levels, but it will also provide the additional boost you require in order to maintain your concentration and find more effective solutions to difficulties. Walking and other aerobic workouts enhance the amount of blood that flows to the brain, which in turn improves cognitive performance and concentration. As a consequence of this, engaging in intermittent bouts of walking during the course of the workday can help you maintain your concentration. Walking can also help you live longer by lowering your risk of developing neurological disorders like dementia. This lowers your overall risk of death.

Walking can become a mindful activity that places an emphasis on the present moment if one focuses their attention on each individual step as they walk. Similar to meditation, mindful walking is a simple practice that can help reduce feelings of worry and produce an overall sense of wellbeing.

Keeping one's focus on the most important task at hand can be of tremendous value in the workplace. Your ability to focus better and maintain your attention for longer can be a driving force behind your professional success, irrespective of the sector in which you now operate. Here are some reasons why maintaining attention at work is beneficial.

Builds momentum: Maintaining concentration on a single task increases the likelihood that it will be finished in a manner that is more productive. Your capacity to complete jobs in a more expedient manner has the potential to encourage you to move on to the next one. Knowing that you are capable of accomplishing things will help you maintain a positive attitude and drive you to work toward reaching your next objective.

Drives up levels of productivity: If you are able to maintain focus throughout the day, you will be able to accomplish a greater number of activities. Eliminating or reducing as many distractions as possible is a fantastic way to stay in the zone and give your brainthe space it needs to comprehend what requires your attention. When you focus the majority of your attention on a single task, youwill likely be able to complete a greater quantity of work.

Helps to relieve tension: You can reduce the amount of stress and anxiety that you're under by remaining focused on the task at hand and boosting the amount of work that you get done. When you limit your attention to just one task at a time, you are able to cross more items off your to-do list and make more room in your work calendar for other activities. Your capacity to channel your energy in productive ways will ensure that you don't get behind on work and that you don't have to scramble to meet deadlines at the eleventh hour.

Produces better quality work: Your capacity for concentrationis one of the most important factors determining your level ofsuccess in the profession. Your ability to generate high-quality work directly correlates to the amount of time and focus you can put into a single project at a given time. Not only will you be ableto complete jobs in a shorter amount of time, but you will also be able to guarantee that they are error-free.

CHAPTER SIXTEEN
Improved Executive Function

During the course of their workdays, people like Truman, Aristotle, Freud, Darwin, and Beethoven all went on lengthy walks. According to Frédéric Gros, a philosophy professor at the Institute of Political Studies, walking is a significant part of the work that the CEOs of LinkedIn, Twitter, and Facebook do. Their companies' CEOs are now following in their footsteps. The intellect can be sharpened, uncertainty and procrastination may be dispelled, goodendorphins can be released, and inspiration and creativity can be encouraged through walking meetings, walking breaks, and even brief walks around the workplace or on a treadmill. Recent research has shown that walking physically modifies the brain, boosting its plasticity and promoting the formation of additional brain cells. This finding is in addition to the abundant evidence that supports the benefits of walking for both the body and the mind. Researchers using epidemiological methods came to the conclusion that walking wards off cognitive decline in the brain. These findings provide credence to a statement that was made by Nietzsche more than a century ago, which is as follows: "All truly great thoughts are conceived by walking. (*Enhance Decision Making and Problem Solving by Walking*, n.d.)

One example that shows how walking can improve executive functions such as planning, decision-making, and problem-solving is the phenomenon of having a walking meeting. As mentioned earlier, great minds, past and present, are upholding the practice of walking to enhance their ability to think through issues at hand.

Meetings have been revolutionized beyond all recognition as a direct result of the rise of remote work and the associated flexibility that comes with it. As a direct result of the widespread adoption of virtual and hybrid meeting formats by businesses, new categories of gatherings are coming into existence. One example of this is holding meetings while walking. Walking meetings, which combine getting some exercise with getting work done, are becoming an increasingly common practice. Participants in a walking meeting go for a stroll together while conducting business, coming up with new ideas, or otherwise going over meeting- related business. It has been demonstrated that this kind of gathering offers a great deal of value, not just to the individual but also to the organization as a whole.

The late Steve Jobs is often cited as the person who popularizedthe practice of walking meetings. He was famous for carrying out significant conversations and gatherings in the neighborhood surrounding Apple's Palo Alto offices while wandering around the area. Jobs thought that he had his most creative moments while walking; therefore, he endeavored to infuse his meetings with the same benefits that he had while walking. Walking meetings are a great way for teams that aren't physically placed together to get thesame boost of enthusiasm that they would get from collocated teams. Thanks to advances in technology, these teams can participate in walking meetings from anywhere in the world.

Walking meetings can take place either inside or outside, and participants can go at their own pace or in groups. They can be especially helpful for sessions in which ideas are generated, problems are solved, or informal check-ins are conducted. In addition, because of the proliferation of remote and hybrid meetings, it is now possible to hold walking meetings online, and participants can join in from wherever they happen to be located inthe world.

Advantages of holding meetings while walking

Increasing opportunities for physical activity: One of the most significant advantages that walking meetings offer is the encouragement of physical exercise. Many people spend most of their workdays seated at a desk, which puts their health at risk because sitting for extended periods of time can be detrimental to our health. Walking meetings provide an opportunity to move around and get some exercise, which can help reduce the risk of health problems such as heart disease, obesity, and diabetes. Walking meetings provide an opportunity to lower the risk of health problems such as heart disease, obesity, and diabetes. To our alarm, remote workers are sitting for longer periods of time than ever before. According to the findings of recent studies, the average human spends more time sitting than sleeping in a single day. In her pioneering TED Talk, author Nilofer Merchant brought attention to this topic as well as the need to hold walking meetings (Sherpany, *How to Run Walking Meetings*, n.d.).

Enhances Cognition: Walking meetings have been shown to be beneficial not only to participants' physical health but also to their cognitive performance and their creative output. According to a number of studies, walking can increase blood flow to the brain, which can help with improved concentration, problem-solving abilities, and decision-making. When applied in a professional situation where employees are expected to be able to think clearly and make snap judgments, this can be an exceptionally beneficial skill to have.

Enhanced dynamics within the team: Another advantage of holding meetings while walking is that they can help strengthen the dynamics of the team. Walking side by side with coworkers might generate a more laid-back and casual atmosphere, which can make it simpler for individuals to open up and discuss their thoughts with one another. This has the potential to improve both communication and collaboration, both of which can eventually lead to improved outcomes for the firm. People who take part in walking meetings are more engaged than those who take part in meetings in general, according to a study that was published in the Harvard Business Review (Sherpany, *How to Run Walking Meetings*, n.d.).

Increases in Productivity: Walking about during meetings provides attendees with a welcome change of scenery as well as a welcome reprieve from the monotony of sitting still for extended periods of time. It has been demonstrated that leading a sedentary lifestyle reduces productivity, while exercising regularly increases productivity. Therefore, maintaining an active lifestyle during the course of the workday is advantageous to performance, and walking meetings are an efficient way to make this happen.

Walking meetings certainly have their benefits, but they also come with a few possible drawbacks. For one thing, it's possible that not everyone would be a good fit for them. People who have trouble moving around, for instance, might not be able to take part in meetings that take place while walking. In addition, the use of walking meetings isn't always recommended for different kinds of gatherings. For instance, if you want to give a presentation or hold a training session, a walking meeting might not be the best structure to use.

How to conduct a walking meeting

Walking meetings are a fantastic way to get some exercise and converse about significant issues relating to work or business at the same time. There are a few crucial aspects that need to be kept in mind in order to operate a successfulwalking meeting, and they are as follows:

- First things first, make sure the meeting is scheduled in advance and that everyone who will be there is aware that it will be a walking meeting. Cedric X. Bryant, president and chief science officer of the American Council on Exercise, is quoted as saying, "Notify meeting attendees in advance so they can dress accordingly and choose a flat path—ideally in a quiet area like a park."

- The next step is to create an agenda for the meeting and ensure that it is followed. Even though walking meetings area fun way to break up the routine of other types of meetings, it is still essential to maintain concentration and get work done during these gatherings. During the course of the meeting, you need to make sure that the conversation stays on topic and does not veer off in other directions.

- To get the most out of a walking meeting, though, you need to be willing to let there be some amount of informality. This will allow participants to completely benefit from the style of the meeting while also allowing them to express their creativity. Therefore, as the leader of the meeting, you need to be willing to ensure that there is structure, but you should also be willing to provide some wiggle room.

- Last but not least, make it a point to get some kind of meeting feedback during your walking meetings. Does your team have success with this structure? What is it exactly that people enjoy about it? Should this be something that comes up at each and every one of your standing meetings?

It is essential to prepare in advance if you want to get the most out of your walking meetings. Ensure that you have a detailed agenda for the meeting and that everyone is aware of what they should anticipate throughout the gathering. You should pick a site that everyone can get to easily and that is secure, and you should also consider the forecast as well as any other potential challenges. Walking meetings are an excellent approach to encouraging physical activity as well as improving creativity. They have the potential to help improve the dynamics of a team, which in turn can lead to improved results for your firm.

CHAPTER SEVENTEEN
Better Blood Sugar Regulation

Your levels of naturally occurring melatonin go up and down throughout the day, much as your blood sugar does at different points in the day. According to the Center for Disease Control and Prevention (CDC), when you eat, your blood sugar levels rise, and your pancreas produces a hormone called insulin in response to the rise in blood sugar. This hormone sends a signal to the body to soak up glucose, which in turn helps lower blood sugar levels. The body uses glucose in one of these three ways:

- Put that sugar to use as fuel right now.

- Those calories are converted into glycogen and stored in the liver for subsequent use.

- It undergoes conversion into fatty acids so that it can be stored as fat in our adipose tissue.

Insulin resistance can throw this process off track or make it more difficult for people who have already been diagnosed with prediabetes or type 2 diabetes. However, whether you already have diabetes or not, it is best to keep your blood sugar levels within a reasonably stable range. This will help you retain sustained energy and lower the likelihood that you may acquire type 2 diabetes in the future.

One of the simplest, most cost-effective, and most reliable ways to assist your body in maintaining a stable level of sugar is to put on your shoes (whether they be sneakers or sandals) and go for a walk. A post-meal walk of as little as two to five minutes may havea big impact on blood sugar levels, and the advantages grow if you take even more steps and make physical activity a regular part of your routine. If you have diabetes, a post-meal walk of as little as two to five minutes may have a substantial influence on blood sugar levels. (*The Best Walking Plan to Help Lower Your Blood Sugar Levels*, 2023)

According to Michele Canon, NASM, CPT, a fitness nutrition specialist, behavioral change coach, and an XPro for Stride Fitness on Xponential in Pasadena, California, the movements your body makes while walking stimulate muscle contractions and blood flow, which helps deliver glucose from outside the muscle cell to inside. Canon is based in Pasadena, California. According to James

S. Skinner, Ph.D., a senior advisor on exercise for the American Council on Exercise and professor emeritus in the department of kinesiology at Indiana University in Bloomington, Indiana, sugar molecules in the blood cannot enter muscles without some sort of "escort," so they must be carried along with the assistance of insulin. Dr. Skinner is a senior advisor on exercise for the American Council on Exercise.

"However, in people who are overweight or who lead a sedentary lifestyle, the quantity of insulin that is required to move sugar into cells increases. Insulin receptors on the surface of the muscle become less responsive as the disease progresses. Blood sugar levels will rise if there is insufficient insulin production", as explained by Skinner. If this scenario is allowed to persist for a significant amount of time, it will inevitably deteriorate, and the individual may eventually develop type 2 diabetes (*The Best Walking Plan to Help Lower Your Blood Sugar Levels*, 2023).

According to Kevin Furlong, DO, a clinical associate professor of endocrinology at Thomas Jefferson University in Philadelphia, the most important factor in maintaining proper blood sugar control isregular physical activity. According to the American Diabetes Association (ADA), getting adequate exercise is just as critical to the management of type 2 diabetes as maintaining a healthy diet, taking prescribed medications, and finding healthy ways to deal with stress. People who had prediabetes and participated in a landmark multicenter research study in 2002 called the Diabetes Prevention Program discovered that their odds of acquiring full- blown diabetes were dramatically lowered if they exercised for 150 minutes per week and lost approximately 7 percent of their body weight. "This has been replicated in other trials since," explains Dr.Furlong (Orenstein & MD, MSPH, 2015).

Walking, which has a "low impact" and is "less likely to injure joints and ligaments," is one of the most beneficial activities that you can perform, according to Furlong. There is no cost involved, and you can perform the activity virtually anywhere. People are encouraged to aim for 10,000 steps per day by a wide variety of health advocates, in addition to a large number of fitness applications and devices. According to Shape Up America!, a nonprofit organization that focuses on obesity and weight control, the average person walks around five miles when they complete ten thousand steps. Karen Kemmis, PT, CDE, a certified diabetes educator with SUNY Upstate Medical University in Syracuse, New York, and a member of the executive board of the American Association of Diabetes Educators, recommends that people with type 2 diabetes who are just starting out not assume that it's all or nothing. She says that a goal of 10,000 steps may be unrealistic for people with type 2 diabetes who are just getting started. Begin on alow scale and gradually increase it.

Kemmis recommends that you buy either an activity tracker or an app for your phone to help you keep track of the number of steps you take and recognize your progress toward your goals, regardlessof how much walking you intend to do (Orenstein & MD, MSPH, 2015).

CHAPTER EIGHTEEN

Deepens Social Interaction

Research is accumulating more and more evidence that having strong social bonds is essential to maintaining healthy brain function. Engaging in social activities can help develop brain networks while also improving attention and memory. Even though you're just laughing and chatting, your mind is actively processing everything that's going on. The benefits of this increased brain activity become apparent over time. Researchers have discovered that those with robust social networks have a lower risk of experiencing cognitive decline in comparison to those who spend the majority of their time by themselves. In fact, the findings of a comprehensive study that involved over 12,000 participants suggest that the risk of dementia in individuals who are socially isolated increases by as much as 40% (Bilodeau, 2021).

As we get older, it can become increasingly challenging to maintain our social connections. Over the course of time, friendships can become strained, and family members are frequently preoccupied with their own lives. "People who were disconnected from others were roughly three times more likely to die during the nine-year study than people with strong social ties," John Robbins recounted in his wonderful book on health and longevity, "Healthy at 100". Beginning in 1965, Lisa F. Berkman and S. Leonard Syme conducted the research in Alameda

County, California. The study included 7,000 men and women.

This significant disparity in survival rates was observed across all demographic categories, including age, gender, health behaviors, and physical health status. In fact, the researchers discovered that "those with close social ties and unhealthful lifestyles (such as smoking, obesity, and lack of exercise) actually lived longer than those with poor social ties but more healthful living habits," Mr.Robbins stated in his summary of the study's findings. On the other hand, he swiftly added, "It goes without saying that those individuals who led healthy lifestyles in addition to having close social ties lived the longest of all" (Bilodeau, 2021).

Researchers in the department of sociology at the University of Texas at Austin, Debra Umberson and Jennifer Karas Montez, cited "consistent and compelling evidence linking a low quantity orquality of social ties with a host of conditions" in a report that was published in 2010 in The Journal of Health and Social Behavior. These conditions include the development and worsening of cardiovascular disease, repeat heart attacks, autoimmune disorders, high blood pressure, cancer, and slowed wound healing. The researchers from Texas made the point that engaging in social activities can improve one's health by having a beneficial effect on the lifestyle choices that people make. For instance, if none of your friends are smokers, you'll have less of a desire to pick up the habit yourself. According to the findings of the study, the adoption of healthy behaviors such as engaging in regular exercise, consuming a balanced diet, and refraining from smoking, excessive weight gain, and abusive use of alcohol and drugs "explains about 40 percent of premature mortality as well as substantial morbidity and disability in the United States". (Brody, 2017)

A lack of social connections can also have a negative impact on mental health. According to the Texas researchers who published their findings, the emotional support that social ties provide helps to lessen the negative effects of stress and can develop "a sense of meaning and purpose in life."

Walking is one of the easiest and most successful methods to connect with other people, and it's been around almost as long as humanity has. Walking provides a one-of-a-kind opportunity to cultivate meaningful social contacts, which can enrich your life in a variety of ways. This is true whether you're ambling through a park, hiking on a nature route, or even making your way through the streets of an urban area.

The power of talking and walking

Conversations might take place in an atmosphere that is more laid-back and casual when walking. As you walk beside someone else and have a conversation, there is something intrinsically relaxing about the experience. It is possible that people will feel less pressured to open up and express themselves if they are not forced to maintain direct eye contact with one another. Conversations that take place while walking often have a more natural flow. The calm cadence of your steps provides a reassuring backdrop for your conversation, which in turn helps to put both you and your walking companion at rest. This may result in conversations that are more genuine and forthright.

The peaceful arms of Mother Nature

The quality of social interactions is improved by walking in natural areas like parks, forests, or along the coastline of a body of water, for example. The peacefulness and splendor of nature can help break the ice between people. A stronger connection and a sense of oneness might develop between you and your strolling buddy if you both take pleasure in the natural beauty of the area. Additionally, spending time in natural settings has been shown to lower feelings of tension and anxiety, creating a mood that is more conducive to discourse. It's as if the peace and quiet of the setting seeps into your interactions, elevating their level of pleasantness and making them more delightful overall.

The Community Connection That Walking Groups Provide

Participating in a walking club or joining a walking group is a great way to mix getting exercise with interacting with other people. Because the members of these organizations tend to share interests and objectives, it is easier to connect with one another and to start new connections among them. A sense of camaraderie and belonging can be gained by going on a walk with a group. Camaraderie and mutual support can be fostered through the shared experience of going for a walk together. These conversations, whether they involve talking about the happenings of the day, exchanging personal anecdotes, or simply enjoying the company of people, have the potential to greatly improve both your sense of connection and your sense of well-being.

Deepening Existing Relationships

The act of walking can also serve as a catalyst for strengthening relationships that already exist. It doesn't matter if you're out on a hike with your family, your significant other, or a group of friends; walking affords the opportunity for quality one-on-one time, which is essential for having meaningful conversations. Walking enables deeper and more meaningful relationships to be made between people in a society where many social encounters are often shallow or hurried. It is an opportunity to catch up with one another, to talk about your ideas and feelings, and to reinforce the links that bind you together.

Mindful Connections

Walking is another activity that may be used to practice mindfulness, which involves bringing one's attention to the here and now as well as one's surroundings. When you walk with a friend or loved one, practicing mindfulness together has the potential to develop a relationship that is both one-of-a-kind and profound. You and your companion are having a thoughtful experience together as you take in all that the stroll has to offer in terms of sights, sounds, and sensations. Because you both have this knowledge, it will be easier for the two of you to appreciate the splendor of the world that surrounds you.

CHAPTER NINETEEN

How to Walk

The beauty of walking lies not only in its accessibility but also inthe myriad places it can be undertaken. From the bustling streetsof urban centers to the tranquil paths winding through lush forests, our world is rich with options for those who wish to harness the power of walking as a means to enhance physical fitness, mental well-being, and a profound connection with nature. As our lives become increasingly hectic and digital, the act of walking provides a respite, allowing us to unplug, unwind, and reconnect with the physical world.

The diversity of walking spaces mirrors the diversity of human interests and lifestyles. For those who crave a serene communion with nature, the meandering trails of parks and the rugged paths ofhiking trails beckon, offering an opportunity to breathe in the earthy scent of the outdoors. In contrast, the rhythmic pulse of citystreets and urban centers serves as a backdrop for brisk walks amid the constant ebb and flow of daily life. Malls, once havens of consumerism, have evolved into unexpected fitness sanctuaries, welcoming early-morning walkers who tread their climate- controlled corridors. Alongside these unconventional paths, college campuses open their quads to both students and the public, inviting exploration on foot amid academic and architectural wonders.

For those with a taste for history, the cobblestone streets of historic districts, lined with centuries-old buildings, hold stories of generations past, offering a cultural and physical journey in one. Alternatively, the gentle rustle of leaves along riverfronts and waterfronts creates a tranquil environment conducive to peaceful strolls. Each walking space offers unique benefits to the walkers who traverse it.

Parks and nature trails

A community's parks and walking paths are two of its most valuable assets. Homes, parks, businesses, and educational institutions are all easily accessible on foot or by bicycle in a neighborhood that has been thoughtfully planned. All members of the community are afforded the opportunity to take advantage of these paths, which are beneficial to both their physical and emotional well-being. A fatigued brain might benefit from walking or sitting in nature, which can help to renew and reinvigorate it. There is a substantial body of data in the field of science that is stillexpanding to support the idea that spending time in nature has beneficial impacts on the quality and quantity of sleep, stress levels, social interactions, memory, attention, creativity, and other areas of mental and cognitive health. Exposure to natural environments may increase working memory, cognitive flexibility, and attentional control, according to a study that was published in Current Directions in Psychological Science in 2019.

Walking in natural settings has been shown to have beneficial effects on health and is sometimes referred to as "green exercise. It can help alleviate stress, and it can also increase one's immune system and mental well-being. Additionally, it has the potential to improve our capacity for concentration and provide greater clarity to our thinking. Studies have also shown that when people have easy access to green spaces, they are more likely to go for walksand engage in other forms of physical activity. To put this in perspective, consider going for a run in the middle of a busy city. Therefore, exercising in a green environment might have several advantages.

Walking around natural areas can have a beneficial effect on one's mood as well as their memory. Following a walk in a natural setting, participants with moderate to severe depression exhibiteda significant improvement in their mood as well as their short- term memory. This is in contrast to when they walked around the streets of a metropolis. It is noteworthy that children diagnosed with ADHD may see an improvement in their attention span after taking a walk in a park as opposed to taking the same amount of time to walk through an urban area. The practice of spending time in natural settings has been shown to both enhance and boost mental sharpness.

According to a study, people who want to start an exercise regimenwill have a better chance of sticking with it if they do their workouts outside rather than at a gym. Studies have shown that individuals who exercise on a regular basis in a natural setting or who are interested in pursuing a type of green exercise are likely to engage in moderate to strenuous activity. On the other hand, people who work out in the fresh air are more likely to want to continue their routine and are more committed to doing so. Those who do their workouts on a treadmill stand in contrast to this. However, if you intend to stroll along a route, you need to give some thought to how you might keep yourself safe. You might wantto think about asking a friend to join you in this endeavor, because the more people there are, the more fun it will be.

Other advantages of engaging in physical activity outside include the following:

Engaging diverse muscle groups and improving coordination, bothof which are essential for maintaining balance when traversing uneven terrain. Vitamin D levels can be increased by spending time in the sun, which is essential for maintaining overall health aswell as strong bones and muscles. Participating in activities outside allows one to be exposed to clean air, sunlight, and a variety of fascinating sights.

Things to think about before you leave are as follows:

- Pick out an outfit that fits the occasion.
- Take precautions to avoid the wind and the sun.

- Verify that the temperature is correct.

- Put on appropriate footwear.

- Keep your senses sharp.

- It is important not to omit the warm-up and stretching.

- Pick the place you want to be.

- Pick an hour of the day to talk.

- Please drink some water.

- Avoid skipping the cool-down and the flexibility drills.

School/College Track

A track is an alternative to walking outside that is convenient, and this applies whether you are a novice or an experienced walker. As long as you are aware of the regulations for safety and conduct yourself in an appropriate manner on the track, it is generally considered to be the safest alternative. Utilizing a track has many benefits, one of which is that it is graduated, allowing you to more accurately assess your progression around the track. If you are walking on a track rather than a natural route, it will be much simpler for you to determine how many steps it will take you to cover one mile. The following table provides a conversion for the distances that you ran around the school track. Check to see how many laps you need to run around the track in order to complete a quarter mile, one mile, and other distances.

Common Distances on a Track	
Meters	Track Equivalent
100	The length of each straightaway, if you are runningsprints; the shortest distance for an outdoor sprint race
200	A half lap around a standard-distance track

400	Approximately a quarter-mile, or one lap around astandard track
600	A half lap followed by one full lap around the track
800	Approximately a half-mile is equal to two laps around the track
1200	Approximately three-quarters of a mile, or three lapsaround the track
1600	Approximately 1 mile, or four laps around the track.

Be sure that when you want to use a school track for your scheduled walks, you check in with the school to see if the time youschedule is free.

Treadmills (at home or in the gym)

A person's cardiovascular health can be greatly improved by performing workouts on a treadmill. As with any piece ofequipment, there is a right way to walk on a treadmill. Avoid making typical blunders by following instructions if you want to get the most out of the time you spend walking on a treadmill. Walking with the correct form and posture is one of the mostimportant things you can do to keep discomfort and strain at bay. Using these guidelines, you will be able to improve the speed and smoothness of your walking as well as the number of calories you burn during moderately intense cardio workouts, which are beneficial to your health and fitness.

If you have a medical condition that alters your posture or makes it difficult for you to walk on a treadmill, you should probably consult a healthcare expert for guidance on how to use a treadmill in a safe manner. This is especially important if your condition makes it difficult for you to walk on a treadmill.

Safety first

The first rule in using any piece of machinery is "safety first", There will be no use using the treadmill or any machinery if the user is not safe. The safety guides are not just there but to be followed. The very first error that people make is getting on a treadmill while it is already traveling at top speed, Instead, make sure to stick to this routine every time you go on the treadmill.

- Start by standing with one foot on each side of the treadmill.

- Locate the stop switch for the emergency exit.

- If you trip while using the treadmill, the safety stop cord should be attached to your body so that it will stop the machine.

- When you first get on the treadmill, set the speed to a modest level.

- After you have boarded, gradually accelerate to the desired level.

- Make sure you are aware of the speed and slowly step onto the moving tread.

This is important because many people who use treadmills end up hurting themselves when the belt unexpectedly starts moving at a fast speed.

Maintain good walking posture.

While on the treadmill, do not start at speeds that will make it necessary for you to hold onto the handrails, unless, of course, you have an underlying condition that affects your stability. It's understandable that you'd like the reassurance of grabbing onto the handrails for stability, but walking or running in such a manner is not a natural way to move. If you are holding onto the handrails, you will not be able to walk with proper posture, nor will you be able to move naturally with a healthy stride and arm motion. If you have a major impairment or issues with your balance, you should continue to use the handrails. However, if you want to acquire appropriate walking posture even if you have to use handrails, you should seek the counsel of a trainer or a physical therapist and discuss it with them.

Look Forward

In the same way that your objective in starting this walk is to move forward, proper walking posture entails keeping your head up and your eyes ahead of you. If you find yourself in need of entertainment while on the treadmill, you may either place your film or reading material so that you are looking straight ahead at it rather than down or up, or you can consider utilizing an MP3 player to listen to music or podcasts so that you can keep your gazeforward the entire time.

When walking on a treadmill with poor posture, you may end up experiencing pain in your lower back, neck, and shoulders. It prevents you from taking full, comprehensive breaths in and out. In addition to this, it encourages people to maintain the poor sitting position that they have developed as a result of spending long periods of time in front of a computer or television. Throughout your activity, give your shoulders a roll backward every few minutes to ensure that you are not hunching them forward.

Walk upright

As you look forward, you should avoid leaning too far forward. The correct way to walk is with an upright stance, without slouching either forward or backward. Before you start walking on the treadmill, you should check your posture for a second to ensure that you are in the ideal walking position. Maintain a neutral spine while you engage the abdominals and keep them engaged. Imaginethat there is a string linked to the very top of your head right now. To lift your upper body off of your hips and into a more vertical position, pull it up toward you. To ensure that your shoulders are not rounded forward, give yourself a backward shoulder roll. Get on the treadmill and start walking as soon as you feel as though you have a straight posture. Remind yourself to maintain this upright posture while you go about your daily activities. Always remember to double-check your posture as you pick up the speed or the incline.

Mind your pace.

Your walk is all about you, so you should not outpace yourself. When you walk with an excessively long stride, your front heel will strike the ground far in front of the rest of your body. In an effort to increase their walking speed, a lot of people do this. If you overstride, there is a greater chance that your foot may touch the front of the treadmill, which may result in you tripping or falling off the machine.

On the other hand, a good and quick walking stride is exactly the opposite. When you push off with your front foot, your front heel should contact the ground close to your torso, but the heel of your back foot should remain on the ground for a longer period of time. This push-off in the back is what will give your walking more speedand power, and it will use your muscles more effectively, allowing you to burn more calories.

At first, it's possible that you'll need to cut down on the length of your stride and just take more rapid strides. The next phase is to start focusing your attention on the sensation of your rear foot and making sure that you are receiving a decent push-off with it with each step. Spend a few minutes of each treadmill session concentrating on this, and keep doing so until it becomes second nature. You will soon be able to walk more quickly and with less effort.

Take walking steps in the right shoe.

The manner in which your foot makes contact with the ground indicates whether or not you are taking a walking step or simply moving in the same manner as any other person would. When you walk, you should land on the heel of your foot while lifting the rest of your forward foot just a little bit off the ground. This is the correct method to take a step. After that, you roll through the step, going from your heel to your toe. As soon as the toe touches the ground, you are already halfway through the following step. At thispoint, the foot that was in front of you is now the foot that is in the back, and you are prepared for the toe to give you a push as you take the next step.

Only if your shoes are flexible will you be able to execute this sequence of heel hit, roll through, and toe push-off. If you are wearing stiff "walking" shoes that are only appropriate for standing, it is impossible for you to roll through a step from your heel to your toes. Instead, the shoe's stiffness compels your foot to land in a flat position. Your walking stride is more akin to a stomping march with flat feet, which suggests that your body may have given up even trying. To remedy it, you need to give some thought to what your feet are doing whenever you go for a walk and give yourself a couple of minutes to do so. Are you making contact with the heel of your foot and rolling through the rest of the step? Are you able to get a push-off with your back foot?

You can focus on a few different things to break this habit, which is helpful. First, imagine that the bottom of your forward foot is exposing itself to the person who is facing you. Then you should focus on keeping the back foot planted for a longer period of time and giving a powerful push-off in order to display the bottom of your shoe to someone who is following behind you. If you are unable to complete this task while wearing the shoes you already own, it is time to upgrade to a pair of walking or running shoes that are more flexible.

Move your arms correctly.

Your arms give you balance during your walk. If you aren't holding onto the railings with both of your hands, what should you do with your arms? Your arms are the most important part of getting good exercise from walking. You can move quicker and burn more calories if you make sure your arm motion is correct. You may be causing some of your shoulder and neck problems by spending all day in front of a computer or TV, but there are things you can do to help rectify them. The trick is that you should only move your legs at a speed that is equal to that of your arms. First, quicken the motion of your arms, and then your legs will quickly catch up to your new pace.

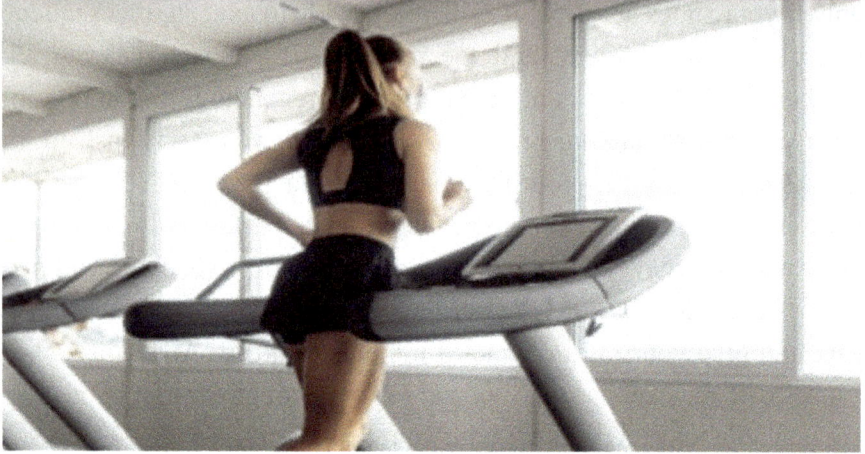

MOVE YOUR ARM CORRECTLY

Know your treadmill.

The treadmill you walk on is your wonderland, and you need to explore all its features to get the most out of it. If you are going to use a treadmill, there are two functions that you absolutely must be familiar with: turning the machine on and turning it off. If, on the other hand, this treadmill is one that you use frequently at the gym or at home, you should spend a few minutes familiarizing yourself with its capabilities so that you can get the most out of it. The majority of treadmills come equipped with an inclination feature. The addition of an incline will provide you with a more challenging cardiovascular workout, which will in turn raise your heart rate. Find out how to modify the elevation on your treadmill and reap the benefits of treadmill incline exercises by consulting the instructions that came with your treadmill. The majority of modern treadmills come equipped with some pre-programmed hill workouts. Walking uphill causes you to burn more calories per mile than walking on flat terrain. According to the American College of Sports Medicine, the number of calories you burn increases by around 12% for every 1% of the grade that you climb (*ACSM's Resource Manual for Guidelines for Exercise Testing and Prescription*, n.d.).

- Speed adjustment: You should be familiar with how to change the speed of the machine and how to speed it up or slow it down while you are using it. After warming up at a slow pace for three to five minutes, you should then accelerate to the pace that you intend to maintain for the remainder of your workout. At the end, take a cool-down walk for three to five minutes at a leisurely pace.

- Heart rate monitor or pulse monitor: Many treadmills come equipped with a pulse meter that may be clipped on or held in a grip. This can provide you with feedback on your heart rate, but if you don't attach it correctly, you might also notice some strange results. A heart rate monitor that is worn around the chest is considered to be more accurate, and many treadmills are designed to connect with such monitors. Check to see if your treadmill offers heart-rate- controlled workouts.

- Personal workout history: Some treadmills record your dataso that you can view your totals and how far you've come over the course of your workouts.

- Pre-programmed workouts: Changing up the routine you doon the treadmill is a wonderful approach to advancing your fitness level. Experiment with the programs that are supplied and see if there are any that you can incorporate into your routine to make it more interesting.

- Apps: Some treadmills allow you to link your workout history to an app, which you can use to accumulate badges, record your workout data, and feed it into other apps.

- Calories burned: Because the number of calories you burn is largely dependent on your weight, you will frequently be asked to enter it. Tell the truth, since if you weigh less, you will have a lower caloric expenditure per mile. However, you should be aware that the calories reported by the treadmill are not always consistent with the numbers you see on your fitness band, etc.

Do not run too fast.

Walk at a pace that is only a little faster than you are capable of maintaining proper posture and form while doing so. Reduce your speed until you achieve a pace that enables you to walk in an appropriate manner. If you feel that you are overstriding, leaning forward, or hunching your shoulders, then you should reduce your speed. Why don't you give running a try? Include some running intervals in your training routine if you feel as though you are not getting a good workout from walking on the treadmill, but your walking form is poor while you are going faster. Running will provide you with additional spikes in your heart rate as well as a shift in your form.

Here is a good example of how you might incorporate intervals of running into your walk-out routine. To warm up, walk or jog at a slow pace for three to five minutes. You should pick up the pace of your walking until you reach a point where you are moving quickly but are still able to walk in the correct manner. Now go into a jog and gradually increase the speed until it is at the same tempo as your jog. Jog for between one and three minutes. You should walk at a brisk speed for the next three to five minutes. Jog for between one and three minutes. Repeat the preceding steps until your workout is complete, and then finish with a cool-down walk of between three and five minutes at a relaxed pace.

Be a better you progressively

If you find yourself getting on the treadmill every day and performing the same old workout, it is probable that you are not making as much progress as you could in terms of improving your fitness. Your body has completely adjusted to the routine that you normally follow, and it will not alter unless you provide it with a reason to do so.

Your workouts need to be varied in terms of intensity, duration, frequency, and/or method of exercise in order for you to acquire increased levels of fitness.

- Intensity: You can increase the difficulty of the workout by either raising the incline or the speed.

- Duration: Increase the amount of time you spend running on the treadmill. If you have been walking for 30 minutes ata time on the treadmill for the past several weeks, you should increase the length of at least one of your weekly sessions to 45 minutes. After two or three weeks, gradually increase the time until you're doing it for an hour.

- Frequency: When you have gotten acclimated to walking on a treadmill, you should be able to do it every day of the week. It is recommended that individuals decrease their exposure to potential health hazards by going for brisk walks of 30 to 60 minutes on most days of the week, for a weekly total of 150 to 300 minutes. If you undertake more strenuous walking sessions on the treadmill and youtypically skip a day, try adding easy walks on the days that you don't walk on the treadmill.

- Variety of Exercise: For a change of pace, you could try going for a run on a treadmill. Alternating between using the stair climber, rowing machine, and exercise bike is an even better way to get in shape. Include activities such as lifting weights, doing circuit training, or doing anything else that you find enjoyable and that gets your body moving innew directions.

The treadmill is one of the most popular ways to get cardio exercise because it eliminates excuses about walking outside in hot, cold, or wet weather. However, in order to obtain all of the fitness and health benefits of utilizing a treadmill, you will need to establish some objectives for yourself and get into the habit of using it on a daily basis.

Walking Outside vs. Walking on a Treadmill: Which Is Best for Your Health?

When it comes to maintaining your health, the one that keeps you the most consistent is always the best choice. Choose an environment that will inspire you to keep moving on a regular basis and go with it. This may require you to begin your workout ata more leisurely pace at first, especially if you are walking on a treadmill and are not accustomed to walking without using the handrails, but in the end, you will have a more effective workout. When deciding whether you want to walk outside or use a treadmill, your objective as well as the conditions of the surrounding area should be an important part of your decision. What is an advantage for one person could not be considered such by another. For instance, if someone plans to go for walks outside but poor weather forces them inside, they can end up walking on a treadmill instead.

Keep in mind that there are a variety of alternative ways to walk indoors, such as going through shopping malls, walking on indoor tracks, or marching in place, in case you would rather walk indoorsor are forced to do so because of bad weather.

CHAPTER TWENTY

How to make Walking Fun and Challenging

⌣⌢

In life, if you want to make something sustainable, make it fun. This principle holds true for even the simplest of activities, like walking. Embracing this philosophy can transform an ordinarydaily routine into an enjoyable and enduring habit. Whether it's a leisurely stroll through a scenic park, a brisk jaunt through a bustling city, or a nature hike that takes you off the beaten path, infusing fun into your walking routine can have remarkable effects on your physical and mental well-being. Sustainable habits are born from a genuine sense of enjoyment. When walking becomes asource of pleasure rather than a chore, it becomes a part of your lifestyle rather than just another item on your to-do list. The integration of fun into your daily walk not only motivates you to stay consistent but also unlocks a world of benefits. From improved fitness and reduced stress to enhanced creativity and a stronger sense of connection with the world around you, making walking enjoyable can profoundly enrich your life.

Below are some ways that you can add a touch of fun to your daily walk to revolutionize your well-being, helping you not only step up your fitness game but also make sustainable changes that will enhance your life in unexpected ways.

Join Challenges

According to the definition provided by the University of Missouri, walking challenges are group activities in which participants work together to achieve a predetermined walking goal or even engage in healthy competition by measuring the number of steps they take each day. A participant in a goal-based walking challenge may set for themselves the objective of covering a certain number of miles (or kilometers, if you use the metric system) of distance during the challenge period (which is typically weekly or monthly), or they may simply set for themselves the objective of taking a certain number of steps during the challenge period. The typical walk is elevated to an entirely new level with walking challenges, which can be an excellent method to inspire individuals to become more physically active. The nicest part about a walking challenge is that it can be done by practically anyone, from complete novices to seasoned veterans.

In the United States, the typical person walks between 3,000 and 4,000 steps per day, which is equivalent to around 1.5 to 2 miles. The majority of walking challenges encourage participants to walk at least 10,000 steps per day. For some perspective, the average individual burns between 30 and 40 calories for every 1,000 steps they take, so for them to take 10,000 steps, it would be equivalent to burning between 300 and 400 calories. Putting this information into the context of the entire daily calorie intake need, the National Health Service (NHS) suggests that women consume 2,000 calories per day and men consume 2,500 calories per day as their recommended daily calorie intake. Therefore, a person who participates in a walking challenge and walks 10,000 steps per day (which burns between 300 and 400 calories) has a good chance of entering the calorie deficit zone, which is necessary in order to lose weight.

If all goes according to plan, a person who participates in a walking challenge will keep up their regular exercise routine of walking even after the challenge is over. Therefore, the objective would be to get people into the habit of walking, which would lead to personal development for each member. According to research published in the European Journal of Social Psychology, the process of developing a new routine might take anywhere from 18 to 254 days. As a result, taking part in a walking challenge that lasts for 30 days is an excellent way to construct and hone the habit of walking among individuals.

How to set up a walking challenge

Walking challenges can be completed solo or with a group of people. If you decide to finish the walking challenges as part of a group, it is recommended that you organize walking groups according to the time of day (for example, in the morning before work, during lunch, in the afternoon, or in the evening after work). This will ensure that everyone gets the most out of the experience. People will be able to exercise at a time that is convenient for them while also participating in group walks. It's possible that having each person complete the walking challenge on their own will still be beneficial; however, the tracking and reporting metrics you use will need to be robust enough so that each person can understand where they stand in relation to the group. Signing up for walking challenges can be as easy as filling out a sign-up form (or forms that are sent around the workplace), or it can be done through any other means that are appropriate for your circumstances. In-house walking competitions are a fun activity for businesses and other organizations to host. Companies that have implemented such a policy have witnessed a reduction inthe amount of money spent on their employees for medical care.

Benefits of the walking challenge:

You should participate in or organize a walking challenge for your team or your employees for several reasons, including the following:

- Walking challenges foster a sense of camaraderie and teamwork among participants by bringing them together to complete a common goal.

- Establishing a foundation for later goal-setting in a high- stakes environment can be accomplished by having a group of people establish goals in a low-stakes environment first.

- This will also help your staff develop healthy habits.

- Improving a group's chemistry can be accomplished by cultivating a highly competitive and goal-oriented environment for the team.

- Your staff will be more engaged in their work thanks to the positive feedback loops that result from a comprehensive walking challenge.

- It's a lot of fun to take on walking challenges!

5K WALKS

The term "5k" is a special way to refer to five kilometers. The term "5k" is typically used to refer to an organized walking or running event with a distance of 5 km, which is approximately 3.1 miles when walked. The events that comprise a 5k might take the form of either highly competitive running meets or more relaxed walkingor running competitions. You can also simply challenge yourself to walk five kilometers at any point in time! Participating in a 5K walk, on the other hand, could provide you with additional motivation to increase your step count. It may appear to be a challenging assignment; nevertheless, all that is required is to walk at a speed of three miles per hour for one hour. Every year, thousands of people set their sights on the objective of walking or running a distance of five kilometers. Participating in some form oforganized event is the most common reason people travel. There are a lot of 5K walks, most of the time for charitable causes but occasionally simply for fun. A 5k event is also the first level of true running competitions, and it is possible that completing one of these races will be the first step toward completing a marathon, whether by running or walking. Going from being a couch potato to walking 5 kilometers in one go is a nice sensation, and it's a great feeling whether you want to take part in a 5k walk or you just want some extra encouragement. The best aspect is that, with a little bit of practice, virtually anyone who is in generally good shape can work their way up to walking 5 kilometers. Participating in a 5K walk is something that anyone is capable of doing.

A brisk walking speed is commonly considered to be at least 3 miles per hour (or 5 kilometers per hour), which indicates that brisk walkers should be able to do a 5k in one hour. Depending on how fast you walk, here is how long it would take you to complete a5-kilometer walk:

- 3 miles per hour: under 1 hour and 62 minutes

- 53 minutes at 3.5 miles per hour

- 47 minutes at 4 miles per hour

There are a lot of informal 5k activities that are entertaining and imaginative, and they are open to everyone, including walkers and runners. There are a lot of different kinds of walks and runs that are exciting that you might try. You have the option of participating in anything from a foam or bubble walk, in which youwill walk through foam that is bubbling, to a costume 5k, or even a zombie run. The vast majority of these competitions welcome walkers in addition to runners, and the primary objective is to havea good time. Find one that is close to you, and you will have a compelling reason to work on increasing your walking stamina so that you can be more active.

Training for a 5K walk

The first step in getting ready to walk a 5K race is to simply train yourself to walk more. The more accustomed your body is to walking, the less of a challenge it will be to walk the 5.1 kilometers that comprise the 5K walking race that you will be participating in. After all, walking one mile can take anywhere from ten to thirty minutes, depending on your pace. If you are able to walk 3.1 miles without stopping, then it will take you between 30 and 90 minutes to walk three miles. This is assuming that you have the stamina to do so. This indicates that your goal for a 5k race should be a walk of one hour, which you may work up to by utilizing tactics for long-distance walking. You can build up to this goal by walking further and further each day.

The further you are able to walk without becoming fatigued, the simpler it will be for you to walk continuously for 60–90 minutes at a time. It will be much simpler for you to cut down on that timeif you walk at a rapid pace if you are already comfortable walking at a faster speed. For a walk of this length, you should generally tryto keep a speed that is quite constant and that you are confident you will be able to keep up for the entirety of the 5.1 kilometers. You could discover that you tire out too soon to be able to completethe entire 5K walk if you walk in intervals. This type of walking is wonderful for short distances but can leave you too exhausted to do longer walks.

Everything that we've covered so far in terms of clothing, schedule, posture, and the correct method of walking is applicable to any entertaining approach that you wish to add to your walking program. Motivating yourself to walk 5 kilometers for a race or simply as a personal milestone can help you walk for longer periods of time, which in turn helps you burn more calories andget in the best shape of your life. Walking consistently for a few weeks should be able to get most healthy people to the finish line of a 5k race without any difficulty. It is sufficient to walk for a bit longer each week until your body has adapted to the increased distance. As you become used to the regularity of training and the excitement of being more fit, you might even find that you are soonable to participate in walking marathons.

TRAINING FOR A 5K WALK

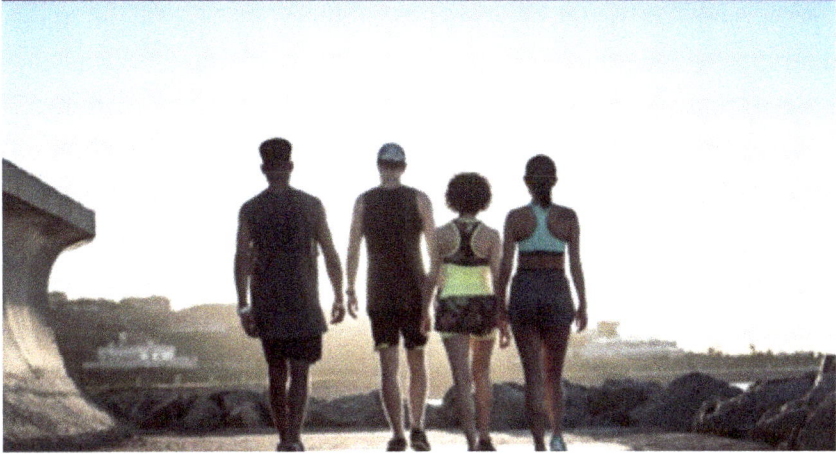

WALKING BUDDY

Walking with a friend not only makes your walks more enjoyable but also encourages you to keep up your daily walking routine. Walking is the best kind of exercise for getting the prescribed thirty minutes of daily activity; therefore, if you want to help a buddy become more active and healthy, walking is the best exercise you can do for them. You will gain an accountability partner who will assist you in reaching your step objectives, and your friend will experience an improvement in their bone and heart health as well as a potential reduction in weight. Walking not only improves your health but also makes you feel better, which in turn can help you feel like you have more of a connection to your friends and family. According to the findings of numerous studies, walking is an excellent kind of physical activity that not only helps you shed extra pounds but also boosts your overall health and bone strength. It will not only make walking that much more fun for you, but it will also provide you with an accountability partner who can assist you in achieving your goals more quickly and push you to strive for even more. Walking with a buddy has numerous advantages, like:

You have an accountability partner. There are going to be days when none of us feel like walking. It could be that something is hurting you, that the weather is less than perfect, that you are in a funk, or that you are simply not in the mood. However, if you have a walking partner, it is much more difficult to blow off obligations. To begin, there is someone to whom you are required to explain your thinking, and even if we are capable of talking ourselves out of a great deal of things, the things we say to ourselves tend to seem less convincing when we have to express them to another person. And it works in both directions. You are able to assist your friend in remaining accountable. And part of being accountable is really getting up and going for a walk.

Joy: Having a walking companion is enjoyable for a number of reasons, not the least of which is the fact that it enables us to see things that we otherwise might not have noticed or to view things that we typically notice through a lens that is new to us. The ability to share in each other's happiness is a significant advantage of going for walks with a friend.

You burn more calories. Do you have any idea how one can reduce their body weight? You let it out with your breath! It's not a myth at all. Therefore, if you walk while conversing with another person, you actually utilize more oxygen than walking andbreathing alone would, which means that you burn more calories as a result of the activity. Walking while conversing is a great way to speed up your weight loss! In addition to that, you get to engage in thought-provoking discourse!

Challenge Yourself: When you have someone to walk with, you are more likely to get out of the house, go a bit further, challenge yourself, and step up the pace. When it comes to generating and overcoming problems, as well as stepping outside of our comfort zones when we feel the need for a little extra motivation, twominds are better than one!

A support system: We all require various forms of assistance, and having a walking companion fulfills all of these requirements admirably. You can stroll while conversing. When you don't feel like moving, you can obtain support from other people. When you're not in the setting you're used to, it's easier to have conversations about various topics. You can seek advice or offer your own, and the topics covered range from walking and walking gear to family, career, and other aspects of life.

What a difference itcould make if you did this on a daily basis!

It's time for some change. Every single one of us is susceptible to falling into the same routine. We go for our customary stroll, which lasts the customary amount of time and is completed at the customary speed. Having a walking partner inspires us to try new things, not only in terms of the route that we take but also in termsof the topics that we discuss, the pace at which we walk, and even our overall disposition for the day. Even when walking, it's easy to fall into a routine. But when you go for a walk with a friend, there are two of you to take into account, which forces you to step outside of your own thoughts for a while. Always a positive development.

Making models: When you walk with another person, you pick up their mannerisms and routines. Possibly walking, stretching, or gaining knowledge about the natural world will do the trick. Perhaps the key is learning how to pay attention to what others have to say. Walking alongside one another can help us improve both as humans and as walkers because our species was designed to learn from one another.

Walk While You Work: Having a meeting while walking is a fantastic way to come up with new ideas, get some exercise, andget away from your desk or computer screen. You may even take a stroll during your lunch break to help clear your mind or solve a problem at work. It's a fantastic opportunity to broaden your professional horizons or take your career to the next level!

Four-Legged Acquaintances for the Trail: A walking partner who has four legs is an excellent choice for a walking companion. What about getting a walking companion for your four-legged companion, though? You can get the same benefits from walking with another dog as you would from having a walking companion for yourself. New things to sniff and discover, improved abilities for walking or training, and the bonding experience of doing something together are all on the agenda. Therefore, you should think about purchasing a walking companion for your dog from time to time.

It's easy to get the healthy lifestyle bug. According to the findings of a study that was conducted at University College London and reported on by the Telegraph, people in partnerships were far more likely to engage in healthy behaviors like exercising more, losing weight, or quitting smoking if their spouse was also active in such healthy behaviors. Having a walking partner not only provides you with someone to talk to about becoming more active but also enables you to trade advice on how to rack up more steps in a day.

Walk in more safety: Your walks can be safer and provide you with a greater sense of security if you walk with a companion. Having a walking partner, particularly if you go late at night or very early in the morning, might provide you with a sense of security. If you are going to go hiking or walking in a remote place, it is imperative that you bring a companion with you in the event that you become disoriented or hurt. Your stroll will be more pleasurable and more likely to be completed if you are certain that you have someone to turn to in the event that something unexpected occurs. If you have pre-existing health concerns, your walking companion may be able to assist you in recognizingpotential signs and providing assistance if it is required.

Keep your walks interesting.Simple is best.

You should make every effort to walk on level ground that is free ofany inclines, declines, or stairs that could make the walk particularly strenuous. Your companion is more likely to continue walking if you make the walks fun for them, at least until they become used to walking for fitness. While you may be focused on walking to burn calories, your friend is more likely to persist with walking if you make the walks entertaining for them.

Keep it to a minimum.

It is likely that you do not know the level of stamina that your friend possesses, so it is best to begin with shorter walks. Find walking routes or sites where you may easily cut your stroll short early or stop and take a break, such as a mall or shopping center, and look for those places.

Always be mindful.

Make an effort to remain conscious of your friend's energy level and how taxing the walk is for them at all times. If it appears that your buddy is having trouble breathing normally, you should recommend that they take a break yourself. This will save your friend from feeling awkward about having to ask to take a break or slow down. If you make the walks enjoyable and fascinating, your companion will soon develop the same addiction to walking that you do. When they arrive, it's possible that your friend will be the one to issue a challenge to you in the form of a vigorous and speedy fitness walk.

Pay attention to the exciting portion.

Instead of focusing on the physical activity aspect of walking when you are just starting out with it as a form of exercise, make walkingpart of an enjoyable day out. Try to organize a walking expedition with a different objective in mind rather than going for a stroll to get your heart rate up for 30 minutes. It can involve going on a stroll with a friend to get some coffee or exploring the sites in the neighborhood. Not only will the activity help you get in your steps, but it will also be a terrific way to show your friends and family how much fun walking can be and to get them into a routineof walking regularly.

Keep a record of your joint progress.

You can keep each other motivated by working together to set goals and keeping track of your overall progress toward those goals. Share the steps you've taken with one another, and if one of you is having trouble, try to encourage the other person or provide them with some advice. Not only will it demonstrate how far the two of you have gone, but it will also be able to monitor the ways inwhich your health has improved and acknowledge both of your accomplishments. Walking does not have to be a competition in which one person emerges victorious. Instead, you should concentrate on becoming better together and accomplishing your fitness objectives.

Facebook Groups

Platforms for social media have fundamentally altered the way in which we interact with one another. Among these, Facebook is the one that stands out as a pioneer because it provides users with access to a broad online community that transcends physical locations. One of the most striking features of Facebook is its capacity to bring together individuals who have hobbies and pursuits in common with one another. In fact, Facebook is not simply a platform for keeping in touch with old pals; it's also a dynamic environment where you may meet people who share the same hobbies, interests, and causes as you do.

The Groups feature on Facebook is one of the key ways that the platform makes it easier for people to connect with others who share their interests and passions. Individuals can come togetherto debate, exchange ideas, and investigate issues of interest to them through the use of Facebook groups, which function as virtual communities. It doesn't matter if you're a foodie, a fitness fanatic, a collector of classic automobiles, or a vintage car enthusiast; there's probably a Facebook group out there for you. There are also walking clubs, of course.

The power of virtual events

In addition to groups, Facebook also provides a variety of virtual events and meetups, which further increases the possibility of connecting with individuals who share your interests. These gatherings may take the form of webinars and workshops, as well as live performances and donations to charitable causes. It doesn't matter if your passion is cooking, painting, or coding; you can participate in virtual events in which professionals and amateurs gather to share their insights and experiences with one another. It's a wonderful opportunity to expand your knowledge and network with others who share your enthusiasm for the things that interest you most in life. When you become a member of a walking group on Facebook, you will have the opportunity to talk about the reasons you want to start walking and the advice that has helped you along the way. Such groups are interested in hearing about both your struggles and your triumphs. You will be able to find a genuine community that will support you on your road toward a healthier way of life. It is a place where you may learn, develop, and connect in ways that were previously inconceivable through the use of Facebook groups, virtual events, and a community that is supportive of one another. Below are some benefits you will get from joining a Facebook walking group:

Motivation and Accountability: Walking groups offer a sense of community as well as accountability, which makes them an excellent source of motivation. The knowledge that other peopleare counting on you to show up for a walk might serve as a powerful incentive for you to maintain your regular walking schedule.

Social Interaction: Joining a walking club is an excellent opportunity to make new friends and interact with other people. It's possible to meet new people, which is very helpful for people who are lonely or isolated and need to feel like they belong somewhere.

Variety of routes: Members of the walking group frequently discuss and recommend new walking paths in addition to their personal favorites. This can make it easier for you to explore new regions and ensure that your excursions remain fascinating.

Safety: Walking in a group can increase your personal safety,which is especially important if you are walking in an unknown location or at an unusual hour, such as early in the morning or late in the evening. There is safety in numbers, and you can watch out for one another if you stick together.

Health Benefits: Walking is an excellent type of exercise, and joining a walking club may encourage you to be more consistent with your physical activity, which may ultimately lead to an improvement in your overall health.

Learning and Sharing: You will have the opportunity to gain knowledge from other members of the group regarding walking skills, walking gear, and ideas for maintaining your motivation to walk. You can also impart some of your own wisdom and expertise to others.

Support and encouragement: Whether you are just beginning your fitness journey or working towards a specific objective, having the support and encouragement of a group may be quite beneficial. Together, you can rejoice in the accomplishment of milestones and get insight into how to tackle difficult situations.

Benefits to Mental Health: It is well recognized that regular exercise, such as walking, can have beneficial impacts on a person's mental health. Participating in a walking group can help you feel happier and relieve tension at the same time.

Themed Walks and Events: Many walking groups host events, competitions, or themed walks for their members. Your normal walking regimen might become more interesting and enjoyable with the addition of these.

Accessibility: Because Facebook walking groups can typically be accessed from any location that has an internet connection, they provide a practical alternative for individuals who might not have access to walking groups in their immediate area.

Free or low cost: Because joining a walking club on Facebook doesn't typically cost anything, it's an easy and inexpensive way to get the benefits of group walking without having to pay any fees.

Inspiration: Observing the development and accomplishments of other participants in the group might motivate you to formulate and carry out your own walking objectives.

WALKING APPS

There is a significant correlation between increased physical activity and lower risk factors for several diseases. Increasing the amount you walk can have a significant impact, and walking apps can help you quantify precisely how much your efforts are paying off. One longer walking session may be preferable to many shorter sessions, depending on the goals that you have set for yourself. According to the findings of a study in which inactive people took either one 60-minute walk per day or two

30-minute walks per day, the longer walk helped enhance strength, while the shorter walks improved quality of life.

The development of mobile technology has radically altered the ways in which we monitor our health and ensure that we get enough exercise. In addition, wearable fitness trackers are becoming increasingly popular. However, because there are so many health apps on the market, it may be difficult to locate the one that best suits your requirements or to determine whether it is worthwhile to use them. Some mobile applications keep track of your walking exercises, displaying information such as your speed, distance, and path. The number of steps you take during the day can be monitored using pedometer apps. Some applications make use of the global positioning system (GPS) and an accelerometer chip in your mobile phone, while others connect to fitness devices like watches. Walking apps are easy-to-use computer programs that may be installed on a mobile device running the iOS or Android operating system and serve the purpose of assisting users in tracking data related to their step count, speed, distance traveled, and other activity-related metrics. Although there are possibilities to acquire premium features, manyof them are available at no cost to users.

Benefits of using walking apps

An excellent point from which to get started: Apps that can assist you in getting started with movement or exercise are a fantastic choice if you're just getting started and aren't quite ready for something more scheduled. They are typically easy to use, yet they will assist you in becoming more motivated.

Advice and suggestions at no cost: In addition to the functions of tracking and goal setting, many applications for fitness and health give users advice. Articles, daily notifications, calendar updates, and even opportunities to join a community of individuals who are also using the app and discussing their experiences are common formats for these health and fitness suggestions.

Easily Reachable and Offering Convenience: In today's high-tech environment, mobile devices such as smartphones, smartwatches, and tablets are almost indispensable. By enabling us to keep track of our health and fitness accomplishments regardless of where we are, mobile applications are now providing us with additional support for enhancing our overall wellness.

Simple in Operation: App developers for smartphones and smartwatches strive to create user interfaces that are intuitive and simple to use so that users can get started using their products as soon as possible. The procedure is straightforward. After downloading a template, you may create a profile that is tailored to your requirements in a reasonably short amount of time and with no effort by answering a few questions about your age, gender, and weight, as well as the many health goals you wish to achieve.

Individually customized and tailored objectives: One of the most valuable aspects of applications for health and fitness is the ability to customize your goals according to your requirements. The goals that an experienced athlete sets for themselves are going to be significantly different from the goals that a novice sets for themselves because of the significant differences in their strength, level of experience, current condition of health, and level of drive. You will be able to input your own personal health information into most of the health and fitness apps, and then you will be provided with guidelines to follow that are tailored to your needs. This is a very convenient feature.

You are able to view and monitor your progress. When it comes to making health and fitness goals, recognizing progress can be one of the most challenging aspects at times. When you first begin a new healthy routine, it may be some time before you see any differences in your appearance. You will be able to observe your own improvement and development through the use of health and fitness applications as you work toward and achieve your objectives. Many individuals find it incredibly motivating to be able to see this information shown visually on an application.

Listening to music or audiobooks

Even for those who walk with the utmost dedication, the repetitive motion of taking one foot after another might become tedious at times. What is the answer? Audio that is interesting. Audio can transform daily walks into engaging adventures that you anxiously await, whether it is your favorite music, an engrossing podcast, an exciting audiobook, or even a language lesson. Audio may do this in a number of different ways. The monotonous nature of walking, despite the numerous advantages it offers, can at times feel like a burden. Your typical walking route may get monotonous due to the sights and sounds that are so familiar to you. It's possible that yourmind will start to stray to things like your daily to-do list or problems, which will lessen the beneficial effects of your walks. This is the point at which transformational audio that is also engaging comes into play as a tool.

The power of music: During walks, music is an ever-present companion for many people. Your disposition can shift almost magically, and you'll feel a surge of energy as a result. Walking faster can be motivated by listening to fast-paced, cheerful music, while listening to slower melodies can induce awareness and calm. Music has the ability to generate strong feelings as well as memories. Your walk might become a voyage through your own history when you listen to old music that takes you back to a specific point in time. Your walks will no longer be boring thanksto the additional dimension of depth and connection that this provides. In addition, the beat of the music might sync up with the pace of your steps, giving the impression that your walking is more rhythmic and coordinated. This synchronization has the potential to improve both your perception of control and your level of happiness while you are walking.

The intrigues of podcasts: The wealth of information, entertainment, and narratives that can be found in podcasts is truly remarkable. There is a podcast out there for everyone, no matter what your interests are— true crime mysteries, science, comedy, or even self-improvement. The fact that they can cater to such a wide variety of interests is one of the things that makes podcasts so appealing. Your daily commute can be transformed into an intellectual and emotional journey simply by listening to a podcast. They offer the possibility of gaining new knowledge, of being exposed to fresh points of view, or of merely being entertained by compelling narratives. Because you become so immersed in the universe that the podcasters have crafted, time flies quickly, and your stroll is anything but boring as a result. Additionally, podcasts contribute to the development of a sense of community. People who listen to podcasts feel linked to the hosts and to other people who listen to the same show because they all share in the experience of learning new things or having a good laugh. This link has the potential to make an individual activity feelmore like a group outing.

The Enchantment of Audiobooks: The world of literature comes to life as you stroll along, thanks to audiobooks. They make it possible for you to experience the joys of reading without the requirement for a secluded spot or a comfortable chair. Audiobooks are especially beneficial for long walks because they may keep a person entertained for several hours. The practiceof listening to an audiobook while going for a stroll paves the way for multitasking. You may improve your health and burn calories by going on exciting adventures, such as solving mysteries or exploring other locations. Moreover, you can do all of this while you are having fun. The antidote to boredom that is provided by a healthy dose of both physical labor and cerebral challenge is not to be underestimated. In addition, narrators frequently inject feelings and expressions into audio books, which enhances the whole experience of listening to a narrative being told. They have the power to make you feel as though you are an integral part of the story and can completely submerge you in the world of the book.

The Edification of Language Learning: Language lessons andother learning materials are a great option for people who want to make their walks more than just enjoyable; they want to make their walks useful as well. Walking is a great way to make productive use of your time, and you can put that to good use by learning a new language or brushing up on your existing language abilities. The acquisition of a language can be accomplished in a more organized fashion by using audio language lessons, which can be obtained via apps or recorded lessons. Walking allows youto improve your listening skills, acquire new vocabulary, and perfect your pronunciation all at the same time, all while getting some much-needed fresh air and exercise. In addition, another type of mental travel is carrying on a conversation in a foreign language while you walk around your neighborhood. Your mind will be enriched and your horizons will be expanded as you listen to stories and discussions in a foreign language, since it will take you to new worlds where people have different points of view.

Overcoming monotony with engaging audio

The answer to that question is that listening to interesting audio breaks up the monotony of walking. The ability to divert attention and keep oneself engaged is where the answer can be found. Audio that is interesting and keeps your attention will pull you into its universe, taking your mind off the monotony of the environment around you. It provides cerebral stimulation and amusement, so turning your stroll into an experience that is not only entertaining but also serves a function When you are listening to something that is utterly compelling, you may not even notice how quickly the minutes turn into hours. You might even find that you look forward to your daily walks, are anxious to continue listening to your audio book, learn about the newest episode of your favorite podcast, or completely submerge yourself in the melodies of your most cherished music. In addition,listening to interesting audio can help you maintain your focus while you're out walking. It is possible that it will help drown out distractions, making it easier for you to be more present and conscious in your motions. This can lead to a greater connection with your environment, which can transform even well-traveled paths into ones that feel fresh and exciting for the first time. Walking while listening to interesting audio can provide a priceless opportunity for isolation and reflection, which is especially valuable in today's society with its nonstop activity and myriad digital distractions.

It enables you to detach yourself from the clamor of everyday life while enabling you to maintain a connection to the outside world through the audio content of your choosing.

Safety notes

Even though listening to interesting audio might make your walks more enjoyable, it is imperative that you put safety first. Take note of the following advice on precautions:

Adjusting the Volume: Make sure the volume is set to a level where you can still hear your surroundings, including any vehicles or pedestrians that are coming up behind you.

Awareness: Maintain vigilance at all times, but especially when approaching crossroads and crossings. It is important to keep yourself from becoming so interested in the audio that you lose awareness of the world around you.

Traffic Rules: Observe and comply with all traffic regulations and signals. Never presume that other road users, especially motorists and bicycles, can see or hear you.

Consider Using Just One Ear: When shopping for headphones, look for models that just cover one ear. You will be able to listen to your audio content while at the same time maintaining awareness of your surroundings.

Your walks have the potential to transform into amazing journeys for both your mind and body if you bring an interesting audio device with you. You may turn every walk into a special and enlightening experience if you choose audio content that is tailoredto your specific preferences, interests, and objectives. Therefore, lace up your walking shoes, put on your headphones or earbuds, and allow the enthralling world of audio to transform daily walks into something that is anything but routine.

CHAPTER TWENTY-ONE

Frequently Asked Questions

In the complicated web of life, questions always come up because we are curious and want to understand and find meaning. We are a curious species, and this easy fact shows how much we all have in common. From the most important to the most mundane, questions guide our search for knowledge and meaning as we go through life. Here are some frequently asked questions about taking a walk as a form of exercise:

How many steps are enough? Does it matter?

The Centers for Disease Control and Prevention (CDC) said that most adults should aim for 10,000 steps per day for overall health, with fewer than 5,000 steps being indicative of a sedentary lifestyle. However, the exact quantity will vary from person to person based on factors such as their age, current exercise level, and health-related objectives (*https://www.cdc.gov/diabetes/prevention/*, n.d.). To establish your own personal baseline, it is a smart idea to count the number of steps you take each day right now. You can then work your way up to the target of 10,000 steps by setting a goal to increase the number of steps you take each day by 1,000 every two weeks. You should probably increase your daily step target if you're already walking more than 10,000 steps per day, if you're fairly active and attempting to lose weight, or if you're aiming to maintain your current weight.

According to Amy Bantham, DrPH, CEO and founder of Move to Live More, a health and fitness consulting company, even though there is not yet enough scientific evidence to support that thisnumber is the ideal target for better health than a lower daily step count, this number actually originated as part of a marketing campaign rather than coming from scientific evidence. One study that was conducted in 2022 and published earlier that year in the journal JAMA Internal Medicine demonstrated that walking more steps each day was incrementally linked to more benefits in terms of reducing the incidence of cancer and heart disease, as well as mortality, up to 10,000 daily steps, at which point the benefit leveled off. The researchers concluded that this association remained true even after reaching this threshold (Pozo Cruz et al., 2023).

Whatever your goal is for a walking workout, the more steps you take, the better. The important thing is that you don't pressure yourself to levels that you cannot sustain and that you check what your present health status can handle.

Can walking maintain your body weight and lower many health risks?

Walking can assist you in preserving a healthy body weight and lower the likelihood that you will become obese. Walking has numerous other positive effects on one's health. It has been proventhat going for an easy stroll every day for thirty minutes can reducethe chances of having a heart attack or stroke. It contributes to the reduction of blood pressure and takes control of your blood sugar levels to lower your likelihood of acquiring type 2 diabetes. It enhances the lipid profile of the blood, improves bone health, and lowers your risk of developing osteoporosis. It enhances your overall sense of health and happiness and decreases the likelihood of getting specific malignancies, including breast and colon cancers, among others.

Is walking exercise?

According to the Centers for Disease Control and Prevention, simply walking as you typically would throughout the day is insufficient if you want to exercise. While more than 145 million people consider walking to be a form of exercise, they are unaware that in order to have a positive impact on their health, they must engage in at least 2 1/2 hours of aerobic activity each week. This means that each week, a total of 150 minutes should be spentwalking briskly for at least 10 minutes at a time. So yes, walking has the potential to be an excellent form of exercise. To reap the health benefits of walking, it is crucial to make sure you are moving sufficiently and at the proper speed.

When compared to wearing shoes, does being barefoot have any advantages when walking?

Walking around barefoot has been shown to improve both one's health and one's level of physical fitness, according to Health Guidance. The concept that underlies this discussion is that, over the course of thousands of years, the human body has developed tooffer us the most effective form of transportation. Despite the fact that the human body evolved over time, people continued to go around barefoot. The development of modern shoes, whichprovide support for your ankle, bridge, and heel, has resulted in a modification in your stride and angle to a point that the body was not built for. The support that you get from shoes can assist in preventing muscle strain and ankle injuries, but it also offers the foot an excessive amount of protection, which you subsequently become accustomed to having as a result of wearing shoes.

When you walk with shoes on, your muscles are not put to work in the way that they are designed to in order to support your body. As a result, you do not achieve the same level of muscular development as when you walk barefoot. This could potentially result in further damage to your ankle and the muscles in the surrounding area. The drawbacks of wearing shoes shed light on the positive elements of going shoeless. When you walk around barefoot, you force the muscles in your feet to work harder in orderto adjust to the varied terrain, which is good for the development of those muscles. Because of this, the muscles in your feet will become stronger, which will make your body more effective overall and make it less likely that you will sustain an injury. In additionto this, you will become more capable of walking for extended periods of time. When you walk barefoot, you put less strain on your feet since you are more effectively utilizing the muscles in your feet; therefore, you will experience less fatigue as you walk.

If you walk around barefoot, you will get more use out of your toes, which is still another advantage of the practice. The structure of your toes is intended to help you adapt to the ground you walk on. When you work out using your toes, you will increase the amount of fat you burn as well as the amount of growth hormone you create, which will lead to increased muscular growth. The additional muscles that you utilize when going barefoot assist in lessening some of the concerns that can come along with walking, such as shin splints, back discomfort, and knee pain. This is because the muscles that are used when walking barefoot are stronger than the muscles that are used when wearing shoes. And if you walk barefoot, you won't have to spend money on walking shoes, and you'll have a lighter step overall. These are just some of the minor benefits you can obtain from being shoeless.

However, in order to avoid cutting yourself on sharp objects, you should only walk barefoot if you are confident and familiar with the trail.

What is good about walking in the morning?

A walk in the wee hours of the morning is an excellent way to kick off the day. Before facing the challenges of the day, it will help you feel happier, soothe your nerves, and relax your mind and body so that you can do so more effectively. In fact, there are several advantages to walking first thing in the morning as opposed to waiting until later in the day. To begin, going for a walk first thing in the morning will give your body the boost of energy it needs to go through the rest of the day. It will wake you up and make you feel rejuvenated, allowing you to face the challenges of the day with confidence. It will put you in a positive mindset, which is essential for one to have in order to achieve success. Going for a walk first thing in the morning helps you get things out of the way for the rest of the day. Taking this approach eliminates the need for you tospend the day coming up with reasons to avoid your workout for the day. Exercising for a short amount of time a few times a week in the afternoon is less likely to turn into a routine that will lead to long-term weight loss than exercising first thing in the morning every day. Walking first thing in the morning can also provide you with positive psychological and social outcomes. People have agreater chance of being available very early in the day before they become caught up in their work for the day. Create a walkinggroup for yourself so that you can enjoy some time with friends while also providing physical benefits to your body. You might even use this time to plan out your day and put yourself in the frame of mind you need to be in order to achieve all of your goals.

I get pain in the front of my legs when walking. What is that?

This common ailment is known as shin splints, and it may be quite uncomfortable. Shin splints are pains in the lower leg that develop as a result of overusing the leg muscles while engaging in physical activity. When people first start a new walking or running routine, one of the most common challenges they face is dealing with this issue. Shin splints, on the other hand, can be easily addressed by self-care measures. Shin splints can be avoided altogether by beginning a new exercise regimen gradually; nevertheless, even if the condition does develop, it is treatable. When you walk with shin splints, you may experience a dull ache or a sharp pain near your tibia. This is how the Mayo Clinic describes the symptoms of shin splints. If you have anterior or posterior shin splints, the pain may be felt more towards the front of the leg, whereas if you have posterior shin splints, the pain may be felt more towards the back of the leg. Shin splints have been known to produce swelling in the area where the discomfort is felt. Discomfort associated with shin splints normally disappears when the affected individual stops moving; however, if the discomfort persists, it may be an indication that a stress fracture is developing. You can avoid getting shin splints in the first place by following a few simple preventative measures, such as the following:

- Maintaining a longer stride length in the back and a shorterstride length in the front

- Putting on shoes that are the right size and have shockabsorbers

- Wearing only shoes with flexible soles and low heels when walking

- You should replace your shoes every 500 kilometers.

- Getting up to temperature before picking up the pace

- "taking a break"

- If you are currently dealing with shin splints, the following are some self-care tips that you may implement to speed up the recovery process:

- Stop what you're doing and rest for a while until the discomfort in your muscles goes away.

- Applying ice to the area and using pain medicines will help minimize any swelling.

- Shin splints can be avoided in the future by warming up the muscles that surround the shins with some stretching and looking into some strengthening activities.

- Arch supports and appropriate footwear should be used at all times during the rehabilitation process.

Don't let shin splints prevent you from getting some exercise by walking. Shin splints are not difficult to get rid of, and while you are recovering from them, you can still participate in activities thatare easy on your shins.

What benefit do I get from incline walking?

Your cardiovascular system is put through an even greater workoutwhen you walk uphill as opposed to walking on a level surface. In addition to this, it makes your lungs breathe more deeply, which boosts the amount of blood that flows to both the lungs and the heart. This is an excellent technique to gain additional exercise without needing to walk any more quickly than usual. By increasing the natural muscle activity in your legs, stomach, and buttocks, walking uphill can help you tone those muscles. Walking uphill causes you to burn more calories during your walk, even though you are not moving any faster or walking for any longer. Additionally, the body makes greater use of fat as a source of fuel and enhances the activity of the leg muscles. For instance, if you weigh 150 pounds and walk a mile at a pace of 25 minutes with no changes in elevation, you will burn around 97 calories for every mile that you walk. On the other hand, you will burn approximately 120 calories if you perform the same walk at an elevation of 4%. The steeper the hill, the more calories you will burn when using the machine. Walking uphill also raises your heart rate, which can only be accomplished by moving at a faster pace. If your objective is to walk rather than run, you can only pick up the pace so much before you start to jog. As a result of the increased workload of your workout—which you'll achieve by walking uphill rather than running, which carries with it the risk of injury—your heart rate will rise.

Is it safe to walk immediately after eating?

According to several urban legends and old wives' tales, it is dangerous to participate in any kind of physical exercise so soon after eating. This might be the case if you want to run a marathon right after eating Thanksgiving dinner, but going for a stroll after a meal is an entirely different story. Taking a walk after a meal is a very different proposition. Even if there are a few things you should keep in mind, it is normally safe to walk after you have eaten. Keep in mind that the kind of food you eat can have an effect on the way you walk, particularly if it makes you feel queasy. Eat a meal that you are confident won't leave you feeling queasy or nauseous if you intend to go for a stroll after you have just finished eating it. This almost certainly implies avoiding foods that are fatty, high in sugar content, or contain a lot of fat. A meal high in sugar will cause your blood sugar to increase, which will result in an energy drop while you are walking. Fatty and oily foods are more likely to make you feel queasy in the stomach. Before going on a stroll, eat the same kinds of light meals that your body is used to eating. If you have a sensitive stomach like I do, it is best to wait at least half an hour after eating before you start your stroll. This will help prevent any discomfort. Even though walking is not a particularly strenuous kind of exercise, it nevertheless has the potential to make you feel queasy since it causes the food in your stomach to move about. If, on the other hand, you are blessed with a stomach that is able to hold its contents well, you should not have any problems going for a stroll right after you have eaten.

Before beginning your meal, it is essential that you give some thought to the kind of walking you intend to perform in order toget your bearings. If you are going to be doing strenuous activity, such as climbing steep hills, you should probably consume foods that are low in calories and fat. It is also possible that you would benefit from eating only half of your meal before going for a walk and saving the other half for after you have completed your walk. In the event that you do wind up eating more than you had planned, it could be a good idea to select a walking route that isless taxing on your body if you have to start straight away.

How do I keep my feet from getting blisters?

Walking frequently puts a person at risk for blisters. It is common for them to appear when you have just begun walking, after you have just changed your shoes, or after you have begun walking for longer distances. Blisters can be quite painful, but there are ways to avoid getting them altogether. You can prevent the majority of blisters by toughening your feet both before and after you go for a walk. To begin, it is essential to locate appropriate footwear in order to avoid developing blisters. Because blisters are created by friction, which occurs when your skin rubs against your shoe, the first step in preventing blisters is to eliminate the friction that causes blisters. Even if there is no shoe that is perfect for every foot, it is important to get shoes that are the proper form and size for your feet. This can make a significant impact. In addition to that, it is essential to break in new shoes before wearing them for a long walk. In order for your shoes to feel comfortable on your feet, they will need to be broken in, which is a slow process that requires you to take your time.

Blisters on the feet are also something that can be avoided by just wearing the appropriate socks. Invest in socks made of synthetic material rather than cotton so that you can benefit from theirability to wick away moisture from your feet. Fabrics made of acrylic and polypropylene are effective at wicking moisture away from the skin and keeping your feet dry. Applying a lubricant to your skin, such as petroleum jelly, will help lessen the amount of friction that occurs between your skin and your shoe. Because of this, rather than having your skin grind against your shoe, it will glide along with it. If you feel a blister beginning to form, place something over the area to protect it. To assist in protecting the blister and halting its progression into a more serious condition, you can apply athletic tape or a bandage to cover the affected area.

How often should I change my walking shoes?

Once you have determined the model of walking shoe that is most comfortable for you, you should feel free to continue with that shoefor as long as it serves you well and only replace it when it wears out. Walking shoes have a finite lifespan due to the fact that with each step you take in them, they suffer a small amount of wear and tear, which shortens their usefulness. The majority of walking shoes should be recycled once they have been worn for 500 miles. In fact, the average pair of athletic shoes is only designed to endurefor roughly 350 miles. If, on the other hand, you walk instead of run, the impact on your shoes will be far lower. Because of this, thelifespan of your shoes may be extended by up to 500 miles; however, it is essential that you do not go beyond this point. You should also take into consideration how much weight you currentlyhave. If you weigh more, it will take longer for your shoes to wear out. If you walk for an average of roughly four hours per week, you should make it a point to replace your shoes every six months atthe very least. If you walk more than this each week, you might consider purchasing new shoes more frequently. Keep in mind thatyour shoes will start to degrade even before you put them on your feet for the first time. Walking shoes are assembled using glue, andthen the glue is allowed to dry. In addition, the padding will lose itseffectiveness over time. Shoes that are currently on sale have typically been in circulation for a considerable amount of time and may provide you with fewer wears before they begin to show signs of wear and tear.

How does walking help the immune system and digestion?

According to Michael Fredericson, MD, a sports medicine physiatrist, doctor, and surgeon at Stanford Medicine, people who walk tend to experience fewer colds because even light exercise boosts their immune system. Walking is a great form of exercise. People who reported exercising five days a week or more (the studyspecifically looked at aerobic exercise but not necessarily just walking) are less likely to be sick with an upper respiratory tract infection (like a common cold) than those who didn't exercise during the week, according to a study that was published in the British Journal of Sports Medicine. The study found that people who didn't exercise during the week were 43 percent more likely tobe sick. According to the findings of the study, people who exercised for as little as 20 minutes at a moderate intensity at least once per week were less likely to become ill (*Homepage | BJSM*, n.d.). (To get at these findings, the researchers tracked whether or not the people who participated in the study became ill over the course of a year.)

According to Fredericson, walking and other forms of exercise raise your heart rate and increase the amount of blood flowing through your body. This, in turn, stimulates the circulation of immune cells throughout the body. It is the increase in blood flow that also gets the digestive tract moving in response to exercise. For example, the results of a short study indicated that going for a walk and drinking water after a meal promoted better "gastric emptying" than the consumption of a liquids such as brandy, aquavit, espresso, or water alone. The researchers behind the studyreferred to this as the process of keeping things moving through the digestive tract.

Conclusion

Henry David Thoreau is credited with saying that "an early morning walk is a blessing for the whole day". As we have seen, walking can bestow a multitude of benefits on our lives, and I sincerely hope that you now have a more profound respect for this exercise, which, despite its apparent simplicity, can have atremendous impact on your well-being. Throughout the course of this book, we have peeled back the layers of scientific research, personal tales, and expert insights that collectively highlight the irrefutable advantages of including walking into our daily routines. We have discovered how this common activity has the power to improve our lives not just psychologically and emotionally but also physically, whether we are doing it on the bustling streets of a city or on the peaceful paths of nature.

When we consider these advantages, it is essential not to forget that the power of walking comes not just from the act of walking itself but also from the intention that we bring to the experience of walking. It doesn't matter if you're going for a quick walk to get your day started, a meditative stroll to clear your mind, or a social walk to connect with the people you care about; the goal behind your feet can magnify the benefits of the activity. In addition, the places we walk, whether they be hectic urban landscapes or tranquil natural settings, each give their own special gifts that contribute to our overall well-being. The natural world urges us to connect with the earth and feel its therapeutic embrace, but the urban landscape may provide opportunities for cultural immersionand people-watching. In this fast-paced and digitally driven society, in which we are frequently linked to screens and trapped behind walls, walking serves to remind us of our innate connectionto the real world around us. It is an invitation to disconnect from the interruptions caused by our electronic devices and the demands of our hectic lives in order to reestablish a connection with our physical selves, our mental faculties, and the natural world that nourishes us. As we get to the end of our walk, I would like to encourage you to go on your own walking expedition if you haven't done so previously. If you make an attempt to incorporate walking into your daily routine, you will most likely discover that the benefits are far more extensive than you initially anticipated. It's possible that you'll find a new favorite walking path, one that takes you to a particular spot that serves as a haven for introspection and revitalization. Keep in mind that the advantages of walking are not dependent on your age or the circumstances of your life. Walking may be a great companion on the path to a healthier and happier life, regardless of your age, level of physical fitness, or when you start your journey toward a healthy lifestyle. Itis a practice that continues for the rest of your life and can change and develop along with you. In conclusion, let us incorporate the advice from this book and the experiences we've gained from walking into our everyday lives. Let us take those initial steps with the knowledge that each one gets us closer to greater health, increased pleasure, and a stronger connection with both ourselves and the world that surrounds us. Let us do so with intention and with joy.

Thank you for your purchase and for taking the time to read this book. Kindly leave an honest review for this book on Amazon and please check out my other books and blogs at **bookpassion.net**.

References

Study finds brain connectivity, memory improves in older adults after walking]. (2023, May 25). Sciencedaily. Retrieved August 15, 2023, from https://www.sciencedaily.com/releases/2023/05/230525135932.htm#:~:t e xt=Summary%3A,the%20onset%20of%20Alzheimer's%20disease.

Put your best foot forward: why walking is good for you. (2014, June 5). The Guardian. http://www.theguardian.com/lifeandstyle/2014/jun/05/best-foot-forward-why-walking-good-for-you

https://www.csun.edu/~vcpsy00h/creativity/define.htm. (n.d.). https://www.csun.edu/~vcpsy00h/creativity/define.htm

Garcia AM, Cognasi TR, Shrestha K, Greene ER. Acute effects of walking on human cerebral blood flow. Submitted to FASEB Experimental Biology 2016 San Diego.

Brand, S., Colledge, F., Ludyga, S., Emmenegger, R., Kalak, N., Bahmani, D. S., Holsboer-Trachsler, E., Pühse, U., & Gerber, M. (2018,March 13). *Acute Bouts of Exercising Improved Mood, Rumination and Social Interaction in Inpatients With Mental Disorders.* PubMed Central(PMC). https://doi.org/10.3389/fpsyg.2018.00249

Social Interaction Is Critical for Mental and Physical Health. (2017, June 12). https://www.nytimes.com. Retrieved August 28, 2023, from https://www.nytimes.com/2017/06/12/well/live/having-friends-is-good-for-you.html

The Best Walking Plan to Help Lower Your Blood Sugar Levels. (2023, January 28). EatingWell.

https://www.eatingwell.com/article/8026946/walking-plan-to-lower-blood-sugar/

Sherpany | How to run walking meetings. (n.d.). Sherpany | How to RunWalking Meetings.
https://www.sherpany.com/en/resources/meeting-management/walking-meetings/

Enhance Decision Making and Problem Solving by Walking. (n.d.). Wharton Executive Education.
https://executiveeducation.wharton.upenn.edu/thought-leadership/wharton-at-work/2018/09/decision-making-and-problem-solving-by-walking/

How to Increase BDNF: 10 Ways to Rescue Your Brain. (2020, September 17). Strong Coffee Company.
https://strongcoffeecompany.com/blogs/strong-words/how-to-increase-bdnf-10-ways-to-rescue-your-brain

Walking this number of steps every day can reduce dementia risk by 50%.(n.d.). TODAY.com.
https://www.today.com/health/aging/walking-to- reduce-dementia-risk-rcna47014

Homepage | BJSM. (n.d.). BJSM. https://bjsm.bmj.com

Pekmezi, D., Jennings, E., & Marcus, B. H. (n.d.). *EVALUATING AND ENHANCING SELF-EFFICACY FOR PHYSICAL ACTIVITY.* PubMed

Central (PMC). https://doi.org/10.1249/FIT.0b013e3181996571

Ahlskog, J. E., Geda, Y. E., Graff-Radford, N. R., & Petersen, R. C. (n.d.). *Physical Exercise as a Preventive or Disease-Modifying Treatmentof Dementia and Brain Aging.* PubMed Central (PMC). https://doi.org/10.4065/mcp.2011.0252

Pozo Cruz, B. D., Ahmadi, M. N., Lee, I. M., & Stamatakis, E. (2023, February 1). *Associations of Daily Steps With Cancer, Cardiovascular Disease, and Mortality.* Prospective Associations of Daily Step Counts and Intensity With Cancer and Cardiovascular Disease Incidence and

Mortality and All-Cause Mortality | Cancer Screening, Prevention, Control | JAMA Internal Medicine | JAMA Network. https://doi.org/10.1001/jamainternmed.2022.4000

The benefits of walking for the brain and more | Walkolution. (2022, July6). WALKOLUTION. https://walkolution.com/blogs/the-walkolution- blog/the-benefits-of-walking-for-the-brain-and-cognitive-function

ACSM's Resource Manual for Guidelines for Exercise Testing and Prescription. (n.d.). Google Books.

https://books.google.com/books/about/ACSM_s_Resource_Manual_for_Guidelines_fo.html?id=HZKFm0VrmhYC

https://www.cdc.gov/diabetes/prevention/. (n.d.). https://www.cdc.gov/diabetes/prevention/

Research Confirms Students Learn More When Walking and Listening toThe Walking Classroom Podcasts. (n.d.). The Walking Classroom. https://www.thewalkingclassroom.org/research/

The New York Times - Breaking News, US News, World News and Videos. (n.d.). The New York Times - Breaking News, US News, WorldNews and Videos. https://www.nytimes.com

https://www.apa.org/news/press/releases/stress/2022/concerned-future-inflation. (n.d.). https://www.apa.org/news/press/releases/stress/2022/concerned-future-inflation

Walking Can Help Relieve Stress. (n.d.). Plone Site. https://www.ag.ndsu.edu/news/newsreleases/2011/aug-8-2011/walking-can-help-relieve-stress

https://www.apa.org/topics/exercise-fitness/stress. (n.d.). https://www.apa.org/topics/exercise-fitness/stress

Orenstein, B. W., & MD, MSPH, J. M. (2015, September 1). *6 Reasons 10,000 Steps a Day Helps Type 2 Diabetes.* EverydayHealth.com.

https://www.everydayhealth.com/hs/type-2-diabetes-care/10k-steps/

Brody, E. (2017, June 12). *Social Interaction Is Critical for Mental and Physical Health.* https://www.nytimes.com. Retrieved August 28, 2023, from https://www.nytimes.com/2017/06/12/well/live/having-friends-is-good-for-you.htmlJane

Getting moving after a stroke. (2019, August 14). Stroke Association. https://www.stroke.org.uk/life-after-stroke/getting-moving-after-stroke

How walking more could make you happier and healthier. (2020, January2). Harper's BAZAAR.

https://www.harpersbazaar.com/uk/beauty/fitness-wellbeing/a30378127/how-walking-more-could-make-you-happier-and-healthier/

Kaplan, D. (2020, May 28). *Surprising Health Benefits of Getting Fresh Air - LIWLI.* Long Island Weight Loss Institute. https://liwli.com/surprising-health-benefits-of-fresh-air/

Upham, B. (2021, July 19). *Want to Take Care of Your Brain? Take a Walk.* EverydayHealth.com. https://www.everydayhealth.com/senior-health/want-to-take-care-of-your-brain-take-a-walk/

[How Walking Can Build Up the Brain]. (2021, July 19). https://www.nytimes.com/2021/07/14/well/move/exercise-walking-brain- memory.html. Retrieved August 15, 2023, from https://www.nytimes.com/2021/07/14/well/move/exercise-walking-brain- memory.html

Bilodeau, K. (2021, September 8). *3 ways to build brain-boosting socialconnections - Harvard Health.* Harvard Health. https://www.health.harvard.edu/blog/3-ways-to-build-brain-boosting-social-connections-202109082585

Asp, K., Migala, J., & RDN, CDCES, L. G. (2022, March 7). *Walking: What It Is, Health Benefits, and Getting Started.* EverydayHealth.com. https://www.everydayhealth.com/fitness/everything-you-need-to-know-about-how-to-make-walking-a-workout/

Pollard, J. (2022, July 13). *Starting a Walking Program: A 12 week plan.*Howdy Health. https://howdyhealth.tamu.edu/starting-a-walking-program-a-12-week-plan/

Rogers,bcbsnc:bio/michelle-rogers, M. (2022, November 14). *Ways walking helps you de-stress | Blue Cross NC.* 8 Ways a Walk Can Help You De-stress | Blue Cross NC. https://www.bluecrossnc.com/blog/healthy-living/fitness/benefits-of-walking#:~:text=Exercise%20increases%20blood%20flow%20and,in%20the%20body's%20stress%20response.

The Best Walking Plan to Help You Reduce Stress. (2023, January 14). EatingWell. https://www.eatingwell.com/article/8024858/walking-plan-to-reduce-stress/

Depressive disorder (depression). (2023, March 31). Depressive Disorder(Depression). https://www.who.int/news-room/fact-sheets/detail/depression

5 Ways Walking Can Boost Your Brain Health. (2023, June 2). AARP. https://www.aarp.org/health/brain-health/info-2023/ways-walking-improves-your-brain.html

www.ingramcontent.com/pod-product-compliance
Lightning Source LLC
Chambersburg PA
CBHW071131280326
41935CB00010B/1178